MW01015848

Health from the Inside Out Series

Healing Comes
from the
HEART

Health & Problem Solving
from the Inside Out

Chuck Spezzano, Ph. D.

Balloonview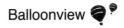

© Chuck Spezzano, Ph. D. 2013

Chuck Spezzano, Ph. D. has asserted the right to be identified as the author of this Work in accordance with the Copyright, Designs and Patents Act 1988.

All rights reserved. No part of this publication may be reproduced, stored in a retrieval system, or transmitted in any form or by any means, electronic, mechanical, photocopying, recording or otherwise, without the prior permission of the copyright owner.

Edited by Eric & Celia Taylor.

Cover design by Guter Punkt, Munich
www.guter_punkt.de

Printed and bound in Great Britain by
CPI Group (UK) Ltd, Croydon, CR0 4YY

ISBN 978-1-907798-39-9

To Janie and Julian

For love and inspired monkey business.

Acknowledgments

I'd like to thank my office support, Charlie Latiolais and Shawna Lum, for their support as I finish these books.

Likewise, my family, my children Chris and J'aime and my wife, Lency, for inspiration and moral support.

To my typist, Sunny Kukahiko, for her truly helpful work.

For Eric Taylor, who studied this manuscript with a fine toothed comb and made many helpful suggestions, making it clearer and easier for all of you.

Lastly, A Course in Miracles and its invaluable teaching over the last thirty-one years.

Contents

Introduction

There are some books that you want to write, some that call you to write them, and others that order you to write them. In the latter case, no matter what your conscious wishes are, you are compelled. This book comes under the latter category. About five years ago, I was guided, nudged and pushed inwardly to write this book. Finally, I was told to muster and was given my marching orders. As a good soldier of the pen, I obeyed.

I take the books I am called to write seriously; they represent a lot of my heart, mind and time. I believe it was the poet, W.S. Merwin, who described poems as times of lost lovemaking. How I invest my time becomes more important to me, especially as I get older. Any book can enthrall me once I dive into it but, as yet, I do not know why this book wanted to be written, beyond the obvious importance of the subject matter. *Why* is not actually something I need to know, yet I am curious. It is my hope, as it is with any author in this field, that this book proves helpful in releasing pain, whether it be physical or emotional. So I offer this book to help release the world from its chains of suffering.

To utilize the mind or spirit to release us from pain, we must first accept responsibility, give up guilt, learn forgiveness and letting go, and discover the gifts hidden by every dark and painful situation.

My own relationship with pain began as a young boy. I remember falling down a stairwell as a child and landing in a sitting position on the last two steps. I had always enjoyed stepping over the head of the stairwell from one room to the next, where the as yet unfinished rooms of the attic lent themselves to all manner of fantasy. I was taking a bigger, farther step than usual over the empty space when suddenly I was sitting on the bottom stair in pain. What could have been quite traumatic turned out to be nothing more than a big, painful thump on the bottom that shook me up, though I was ambulanced to the hospital just in case.

What was worse for me than my own pain was the suffering of my family. I have pulled from repressed memory details of when I fell out of the car at eighteen months old. My parents had finished their first major fight that I can remember. My father had left the house to calm the air, taking my sister and me with him in the car. We were frightened and jostling to get close to my father in the front seat, so he banished us to the back seat in order to drive more safely. Angry at being put in the back, I willfully broke one of the rules of the car: DON'T LEAN AGAINST THE DOOR. As we drove out of the driveway, the door behind the driver's seat which I was leaning against yawned open and I fell out. I bounced a couple of times and rolled into the ditch alongside our driveway. I picked myself up, took the couple of steps to the top of the ditch and was running to my father, yelling, "Daddy, Daddy. I'm OK."

My father had braked and jumped out of the car. I saw a stricken look on his face because he thought I had rolled under the car as he turned out of the driveway. I have never again seen such a look of stunned grief and horror.

There were numerous other times as a boy when I witnessed my parents fighting and the immense pain that they, my brother, sisters and I were in. I knew that my parents loved each other but somehow it wasn't enough. It was then that I vowed that I would do whatever it took to get people out of pain.

There are, of course, many ways to do that but my path was the path of healing, beginning with psychology. As I moved deeper into the mind I studied with healers and psychics, and then moved further into metaphysics and spirituality. In the late 1970's I attended talks by W. Brugh Joy, M.D. and Paul Brennan, M.D. speaking of Wholistic Health. In 1979, I was working with Katie, a close friend who had a supposedly incurable cancer. During one workshop which we both attended, her rugby ball-size tumor shrank to the size of a softball. It still surrounded a major artery and because of this was considered inoperable, but she was well on her way to complete remission.

During that time, Katie had told me the story of her older son who, in a motorcycle accident, had slid 110 feet across the highway on his face, crushing part of his forehead and one eye socket. This eye had been badly damaged by bone fragments, and turned milky white as the pupil had turned up into the socket. This was only part of the extensive damage that he sustained. My friend called in every favor she had, and healers from a tri-state area and from Mexico began pouring in to the hospital, keeping half hour vigils around the clock for three days. During that time, Katie never once left her son's room. When the doctor tried to tell her that her son was blind in one eye, had possible brain damage, etc. she refused to listen. When the doctor examined her son's eye and forehead after the healing vigil, the bone fragments in his eye had dissolved, his bones had healed, he had recovered his sight and there was no evidence of brain damage. The doctor declared it a miracle.

By working with Katie on her cancer, I got my first hands-on practice of working with catastrophic illness. By 1982, I was one of the faculty at the Tubb Holistic Health Center teaching two courses: The Psycho-Dynamics of Catastrophic Illness, and Healing Relationships, which was about the key impact of relationships on health. These courses were experiential as well as informational. The students, who were mostly healing professionals, had a chance to deal with potential issues before they surfaced.

Another extreme experience of pain came when I was twenty-three from my jealousy, possessiveness and heartbreak with my first serious girlfriend. I had only been out of the seminary for just over two years. My girlfriend, who was older by four years, was at the far end of the independent-dependent continuum having been in a number of relationships. I was sunk by becoming so dependent on her. Her independence culminated in her sleeping with someone else. This was devastating to me, shattering my dreams of marriage and a future life together. It was enough to turn me from deep dependence over to an independent position, no longer valuing the relationship or my partner as much.

Over the years, as I worked with my own heartbreaks and those of others, I came to see the many levels of issues that were going on and which led to my first relationship heartbreaks. I recognized especially the replay of old patterns, how I had set them up in the first place and what my purpose had been in having them. Like almost everyone else, I relegated all of this to the subconscious mind, because we would rather be victims and hide the many varied dynamics that go into the victim stance than be that aware and powerful.

Then came my near death experience playing American football the night before I was to leave for San Diego to begin my doctoral program. One of my favorite things in football was to block punts. I quickly shot past the defensive tackle and dove over the halfback in front of the punter. As I was the only one to make it through the line, the other halfback came over and dove through the air to stop me. Naturally, I had tightened my stomach to take the hit from the halfback beneath me. But when I was blindsided by the other hit, coming in mid-air on the side of my helmet, I relaxed and took the hit to my stomach full on. While I still managed to block the punt, I went flying through the air and landed on my elbow, splitting it. I was hurt more than I'd ever been hurt. I had the wind knocked out of me, couldn't breathe and the elbow on which I had landed hurt terribly. I was dizzy and disoriented, and later found out I had a concussion from the hit on my temple. I knew that if I stayed seconds longer lying on the ground, they would send the ambulance out for me, so I pushed myself onto my hands and knees and said to myself, "Get up, you Pussy, and go play football."

I managed to get up and half-limp, half lope off the field. Later that night, I traveled the traditional corridor that occurs in near death experiences. In a workshop about four and a half years later, I intuitively understood why all this had occurred. A few days later, in the next five day intensive workshop, all of the physical pain that I had suppressed came out in a rush. Everyone attending the workshop supported me as paroxysms of emotional pain erupted out of me. Finally, after three hours, they left me in the hands of some staff members to get on with the workshop. In the end, I cried for five hours straight.

It had taken a lot of energy to defend against such pain, and a lot of energy was tied up in the pain itself. Afterwards, I felt at a whole new level of openness and renewal. In the end, I was grateful to have this release and the new flow it provided in my life. My old football tactic of suppressing the pain hadn't exactly been in my best interest. Over the years, I had done foolish things such as playing one season with broken thumbs before I finally had them x-rayed, or not quitting till the end of our practice session when I suffered a broken ankle. Afterwards, the pain became so unbearable as to send me to hospital for x-rays and a cast. In football, I would take the pain, but I was so concentrated on the game itself not much of it got through. Of course, when my mind wasn't on football, the pain commanded my attention.

It is time to have peace instead of pain. While in some survival and physical activities it may be helpful to suppress the pain, it is definitely not helpful otherwise. I was always embarrassed by my pain and suffering. Maybe it was all the times I had to walk past our neighbors' houses as my parents fought, or maybe it was just my predilection, for keeping a strong front, but I always tried to hide my pain as best I could until the pain **made** me feel it. I look back on my life and the emotional pain was always so much worse for me than the physical. I could tell you many more stories of the physical and emotional pain I suffered, but in my case it just begins to repeat itself. I look back on my life and see how foolish and unnecessary it all was.

When I came to write this book I wanted to work with underlying principles that could be used to deal with all pain, whether physical or emotional. When I reached a certain point in the writing, I found that I had exceeded the length of a book and that I was actually writing not just a book but a series of books on healing pain. This is the first of that series. Also, this book is meant to be a form of both healing and study. It is for this reason that certain principles are repeated from time to time, so some of the more spiritual and deep mind principles can be examined and reflected on in different ways at different times.

While this book has been centered around the topic of pain, it can easily be extrapolated for illness as the psychological and spiritual principles are the same.

So I wish you Godspeed in travelling through whatever form of pain you are in. May all of your life lessons be learned with ease and deftness.

Chuck Spezzano
Hawai'i 2009

Lessons

Lesson 1 - Pain is Resistance

The more we resist something, the more painful it is. It is impossible for us to have pain unless there is something that we are pushing away from. This is one of the first lessons taught in a number of chronic pain institutes in North America – how not to resist the pain. This alone has had great effect in reducing much of the suffering. Physical and emotional pain have similar dynamics in this regard. If we are resisting something and trying to push it away, to that extent we are suffering.

Therefore, the more we learn to accept everything in our lives, the less pain we experience. When we fight, we fight against something. Fighting against something is a hidden way of fighting against someone. When we are in physical pain, some emotional pain about this fight has been suppressed or repressed, which makes it impossible to resolve because we have pushed it out of awareness. We do not want to deal with the emotions or the conflict. Thus, while trying to defend ourselves against pain by hiding it, we end up imprisoning ourselves in it.

Just today, I was working with someone on one of their chronic family problems, helping them open their heart, feel the feeling, and embrace the gift that was the antidote to the pattern. It was a very powerful exercise, but it took less than fifteen minutes. Afterwards, some chronic back pain the woman had been experiencing, and spending a lot of money to try to remedy, disappeared.

Today, practice acceptance. You don't have to like what is going on, but if you fight it, it will take infinitely longer to get through and you will feel a lot worse in the meantime. With acceptance comes the next step, and that is the way to freedom. Continuous acceptance creates flow.

Let it be. Accept what is. When you accept what is, you'll graduate to the next step. Accept everything today. Remember the Buddha's dictum to reach enlightenment: desire nothing (no deluding desires) and resist nothing (only blessing what is). While most people speak of the first dictum as the way to enlightenment, they forget all about resisting nothing at their own peril. Today, acceptance is the answer. Accept everything in your life now. Review your life for what still hurts and feels bad. Your acceptance will move things forward for you so that you are no longer imprisoned in a painful history. Make acceptance a way of life for you.

Lesson 2 - *Acceptance*

Acceptance heals hurt. It heals the resistance that causes or exacerbates the pain. When you accept, it allows you to move forward in the flow because what you accept, you naturally let go of.

Recently in a private coaching session, I worked with an attractive young Hawaiian woman in her 30's who had been without a relationship for many years. I asked her to present the greatest pain in her life. She presented the story of an old flame with whom she was still in love. There had been great drama and a triangle relationship until finally he quit, leaving her pregnant and penniless. Later, she lost the pregnancy but had held on to him, never fully dealing with all the aspects of her losses. As a result, she had never moved on enough to be available for another relationship. As she talked about her past, all of the old pain and neediness that she had buried under her independent demeanor bubbled to the surface.

I asked her to imagine her old love across the room, far enough away for her to feel the distance was emotionally right. Using the acceptance principle, I then helped her to let go and move forward. At each step in the exercise, I intuitively felt into this woman to sense what she was resisting, what was at the very root of the emotional pain. I then asked her to accept what she was resisting that was causing her feelings of hurt and rejection. When she was willing to accept instead of resist each of these things, her pain was alleviated. I asked her if she could accept the fact that she was still in pain. When she replied, "Yes," I asked her to take a step forward, not only in the room, but also in her life. Next, I asked her if she could accept her hurt feelings. She said, "Yes," and took another step forward. I asked her if she could accept that she had lost the baby. "Yes," she said, "now, I finally can at this point." I asked her if she felt any better and she replied, "Yes, quite a bit!"

I then asked her if she could accept the fact that she still loved her old boyfriend even though she did not have him. She replied, "Yes," and took another step forward. Each step in acceptance relieved her of a painful burden that she had been carrying for a long time, but had been pretending was not even there. I asked her if she could accept how closed she was to a new relationship and how she had compensated to cover up her pain.

"Yes," she said, "I can see and accept that."

I next asked her if she could accept the fact that she had gotten herself into this mess.

"Yes," she said and stepped forward.

Her greatest fear was that she would always be alone. Of course, her fear had brought this very thing about, and she had actually been alone since the breakup many years earlier. I then asked her if she could accept being alone forever.

She said, "Yes."

Her acceptance allowed her to resist no longer. Paradoxically, it was only then that emotionally she began to move forward in a new openness for partnership once more. Some of the many things she was asked to accept that morning were a challenge for her because the emotional pattern went back not only to her boyfriend, but also to her childhood. Yet, with support, her own determination and the grace that was present in the room, she was highly motivated and willing to move forward once again.

I asked her if she could accept all of her heartbreak and suffering since the breakup.

"Yes," she said, once again stepping forward. I asked her if she could accept the many years she had wasted in her life, refusing to let go.

"Yes," she replied and took another step forward. I then asked her if she was ready to open herself to a new love. With an enthusiastic "Yes," she stepped forward, imaginatively embracing and letting go of her old love. It was through her acceptance that she was finally able to feel equal to "her old love" and to let go of him. She finally felt that she had reached a whole new stage in her life.

Acceptance provided an easy way forward for the resolution of her depression, holding on, being stuck, disassociation, and her hidden pain.

Now it is time to examine your life for anything that hurts, feels like heartbreak or defeat. Accept not only the event, but also everything around this event. In this way you can finally free yourself from the pain, and let yourself go forward in your life once more.

Acceptance Exercise

You could actually do this exercise by yourself. Find an area where you feel hurt or defeated. This is a good sign that there is something you need to accept. Imagine a place in your house that would represent a whole new level for you. Now, go as far away from that place as feels right to you. At each step, ask yourself what you are resisting specifically in the problem you have chosen. As you accept each thing, you can step forward. Remember the alternative to not accepting any particular step is to remain stuck there. This sets you up for depression and a heartbreak-defeat-revenge pattern. Naturally, you will try to cover this up with dissociation and control, and it will not be pretty. Acceptance does not mean you have to like something, but it does mean that you are willing to let it be as it is, without resisting it. Acceptance brings peace. Acceptance moves you forward.

Lesson 3 – Pain Is Healed Through Your Gifts

I recently worked with a young man who had come to the workshop with his wife to improve their relationship. He was in emotional pain because he felt he did not understand women. He was the focus person in the workshop and chose to work on this problem. As we worked, we found two layers of conflict. The first was a domination-submission conflict that he felt he fell into with women. He had played both sides of the conflict and, as we talked, he realized both sides of the conflict came from fear. One part of him wanted tenderness and intimacy and this was in conflict with the part of him that wanted to be independent and always do things his own way.

As we were examining the conflict for the gift it was defending, it became evident that the young man had the heart of a poet. Yet, he was afraid to experience the amount of feeling love and poetry bring. It soon became clear to him how much he had been resisting his gift of poetry and love for women in general. His conflict was just a way for him to avoid losing control, as one does in creativity or falling in love. As we talked, he became willing to birth his poetic gift. As he surrendered more and more into embracing poetry, he felt his heart opening. He was able to cross the room to his wife, energetically sharing his heart-opening gift that rendered him so beautifully tender. By the time he reached his wife, the feeling of intimacy trembled throughout the room. When husband and wife finally embraced, many of the participants were crying for the delicate sweetness that was present.

Any painful situation that you are in is there because, at one level, you are afraid of a certain gift that you are hiding. Take some time to dwell on what gift your pain may be hiding. You can discover it through reason or intuition. When you realize what the gift is, embrace it until it is finally yours and share it energetically with someone. If it doesn't resolve the whole issue, there's yet another gift waiting for you.

Lesson 4 – Ask That

In *A Course of Miracles*, it states that when we want healing we should ask the Holy Spirit, or Universal Inspiration as It is named in its original text, not to get rid of our symptoms, but to remove the underlying fear. It is fear that is ultimately at the root of every illness.

I learned about fear as a core dynamic almost twenty-five years ago. I once had a woman come to my office with a serious precancerous condition. All indicators pointed to the fact that she had cervical cancer, so that when she had exploratory surgery in four days time, it would most likely be radical surgery. Because of our combined schedules, we were only able to get together for three sessions of two hours each before the surgery. As it turned out, this was enough. After the first hour of talking with her, because of the short amount of time before her operation I decided just to focus on healing her fear. So, we spent the rest of the time in her sessions healing her fear. While we went back to the roots of her fear, we dealt mostly with the fear she had in regard to the next chapter in her life, and fear about her purpose.

I demonstrated to her that fear was the way she judged and attacked the future. This fear stemmed from what she'd experienced in her past and projected into her future. We cleaned up a lot of her past so that, as she gazed toward her future, she saw she could do so with confidence. We also concentrated on her living in the present moment to escape fear, which always comes about when we try to live in the future. We worked on building her trust and manifesting positively for the next stage in her life. Lastly we worked on cleaning up her attack thoughts which are another major cause of fear.

The day after our third session she had her operation but all signs of the precancerous condition had disappeared.

I realized twenty-five years ago that every health problem was a fear problem. At one level, fear was a way to stop us from stepping forward to the next stage in our lives. We don't have confidence for the next step because of our fear, and so we need something to delay and distract us from going forward. It then takes us as long to heal the physical problem as it does for us to gain confidence and get over our fear of the next step. Paradoxically, when we take the next step courageously, the confidence to handle what comes next awaits us. *The next step is always better.* It provides the answer to the current emotional conflict that is disguised as a physical problem. We can heal the fear that is stopping us from going forward by simply going forward.

Maybe it's time to ask Universal Inspiration to remove the fear that is causing our physical symptoms and that keeps us back from our next step.

Lesson 5 – Only Perception

One of my favorite quotes from *A Course in Miracles* is, "Only perception, not the body, can be sick because only perception can be wrong." To me this line shows that it is our conflicts, pain, and emotional poison inside that makes us ill, that makes us misperceive. As healing has been a way of life for me, I recognize how layer after layer comes up for healing as we progress in life. If we do not heal ourselves then the lessons back up and can be easily displaced on the body as a result. There is a line in *A Course in Miracles* that states that the Holy Spirit has set up a curriculum for us. When something looks negative, we can use it to realize that there is someone or something we need to forgive outside ourselves, and *give-forth to*, rather than judge and withdraw. When something appears negative we also need to forgive ourselves.

Once we learn a certain lesson, our life improves and then the next lesson is brought to us. These are lessons that our soul wants us to learn in this life and this is one of the best ways to spend our life. When there are lessons we have resisted or refused to learn, our conflicts are denied but not avoided. This can make us ill, or lead to greater and greater mishaps in our lives as our soul attempts to get us to pay attention and to heal what is troubling us. When lessons are avoided they become trials.

All of us have issues. There is not one of us that doesn't have something on our plate to deal with in our lives. There is not one of us that doesn't have some niggling physical issue. It is important not to use our physical problems as a distraction to keep us away from the healing that would do us the most good, which is the healing of emotional issues.

At times we need to be motivated to deal with certain emotional issues as these are full of pain and fear. This is why we have avoided them. It is important that we deal with what we have buried, because what we have buried won't go away if we don't. It takes courage to deal with our conflicts. No one wants to feel pain, unless they are misguided. But it is only perception that can make the body sick "because only perception can be wrong." If we are sick, we are looking at someone, something or ourselves in a mistaken fashion.

Here are a few tips on correcting wrong perception that I remind myself of, both personally and in my healing work:

If there is anger, pain, or fear, there is a mistaken perception. It is judgment that causes all of this discomfort. There are many ways to correct perception, and the judgment it comes from, but the first step is to realize that it needs to be corrected. Every negative perception of others reflects both a misperception and an attack on ourselves and God. There is a misperception when any person or situation looks negative to us. We choose to misperceive by judgment, which is an attack. Our judgment imprisons others, ourselves and locks the situation in the way we have judged it. Our judgment doesn't allow healing to unfold.

Instead of judging, we could bless. Judgment closes a situation and we become right and righteous about how we see things. When we judge something we judge ourselves. We are then in sacrifice because of how the scene appears to us. We suffer both because of how we have judged the scene and how we have judged ourselves.

The quickest way to heal a problem or misperception, once it is recognized as a mistake, is to turn it over to Universal Inspiration for correction. *A Course in Miracles* states that if we have a problem that we really want to be healed, turn it over to the Holy Spirit.

So examine what seems negative to you in your present circumstance and hand it over. Then examine your past and turn that over to a Power greater than yourself, a Power that is only looking to help.

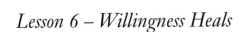

Lesson 6 – Willingness Heals

At the root of every problem, including physical problems, there is fear. It is the fear that comes from judgment and attacks thoughts. It is fear that comes from feeling we cannot complete our purpose, and so we seek problems as a delay. There is fear that comes from our being frightened by our very selves, fear that comes of being frightened of our gifts and our destiny. We are frightened of love and of God, Who is Love. We are frightened of sex, abundance, success, and intimacy. We are frightened of our mistakes, failure, loss, illness, suffering, death, scarcity, and lack of any kind. We are frightened of joy. We are scared of the dark and "our very shadows." We are frightened of fear itself. All this fear paralyzes us, freezing us from going forward to a new level. Yet as we reach each step, a new confidence awaits us. With each new step, there is greater bonding with those around us, and less conflict within us. Stepping forward brings greater giftedness and flow, and there is one less problem.

Willingness cuts through fear. It takes us to the next step. It resolves the resistance that the conflict has brought about. The conflict is the result of a split mind. It has created a problem that stops us from going forward. But willingness does not get caught up in the symptoms of the problem, no matter how distracting they are. Our willingness gives us confidence to see what the next step brings. It allows life to come to us at the next level. This always brings a better connection with inspiration and with Heaven.

Fear is an illusion, but it can be a deadly one. The bottom line is that every grievance with another uses judgment and attack so that "we" don't have to face our fear of going forward, or our life purpose.

Today, practice willingness for all of your physical problems. Today, ask for willingness. If you are too frightened to be willing, all you need to help heal yourself is the willingness to be willing. When you're in a part of your life that is difficult or the root of the problem is the unconscious, it may seem like things are getting worse. Notice, closely, the effect willingness has even if your situation seems to get worse. If you are aware, you will notice the momentary relief because you have moved forward before the next, deeper level brings up the bad feeling again. If you notice this occurring, you simply choose willingness as many times as it takes to get out of the dark territory you are in and onto the next and better stage.

Lesson 7 – The Willingness to Have the Answer

Funny as it seems, we are frightened to have the answer to our problems. I can say this with some authority after many years of helping myself and others through problems.

The answer would free us, but we are frightened of freedom.

The answer would make us happy, but we are frightened of being happy.

The answer would give us blessed change, but we are frightened of change.

The answer would give us more power, but we are frightened of power.

The answer would help us be more truly ourselves, but we are frightened of ourselves.

The answer would get rid of the need for excuses, but we hold onto our excuses.

All of this is our investment in our ego, which is trying to support its beliefs and its way of doing things. This does not bode well for partnership or intimacy, except at best in limited doses, because our ego is made up of fear, the opposite of love. So, while the ego promises to help us contain the fear in order to make itself needed, the ego is not about to get rid of one of its main components. Freud was right. The ego is just interested in homeostasis, with emphasis on the stasis. It is built on the status quo. To change would be to give up some of its control.

The answer is within us. Heaven has guaranteed the answer to every problem. We have been promised that if we seek, we shall find. If we knock, the door will be opened to us. Unfortunately, we listen to our ego, which always has a glib answer, and it is always an answer that will sooner or later lead to further problems and greater delay.

We go to retreats to recollect, remember, and find the answers within us. We go on vision quests to seek the way forward. We meditate to quieten and open our minds. Yet, it is our willingness to have the answer that is the key. When our willingness is stronger than our fear, the answer appears to us. When the answer becomes all that our heart desires, the answer will be there. When there is enough confidence, joining, or love, our answer appears. Our answer will change us and the world around us for the better. Vision then moves us forward in leaps. Our gifts and our destiny wait on us to make our lives and the world a better place.

Today, **want** the answer. Be willing to change and grow. Invest in your soul, your true self. Give up the ego and its fear-colored glossary that it uses to define the world. The answer awaits you. Want it. It's the way out of your present situation. It is the way forward.

Lesson 8 – The Smart Horse

Confucius stated in the I-Ching that the smart horse moves at the shadow of the whip. Pain is an indicator. It states that the whip has fallen. It is a sign that something is wrong. A mistake has been made that leads to pain. I have found that to be the case with physical pain, which comes about when some form of emotional pain, conflict, or judgment has been displaced on the body. Emotional pain stems from a mistake in thinking, beliefs, or choices. It is the result of some experience. It is both the mistaken response to that experience and the deeper mistaken beliefs and choices that led to that experience to begin with.

If we have not corrected a problem from the past, it becomes acute and, as a result, emotional pain leads to physical pain. But when pain does occur, we can follow the thread of dark emotion inside to where the mistake began and correct it there. Sometimes it seems to come from something recent but, typically, the pain is the end of a cumulative pattern that has brought about the present problem and its incumbent discomfort.

Let us be the smart horse and recognize the signals we receive to correct our thinking, end our judgments, and create joining. Otherwise, the separation will lead to emotional and physical pain. It is helpful to examine where we are unwilling, harbor righteous indignation, are stubborn, or even incorrigible. It shows places where we are unwilling to change or grow. If we willingly give up the place where we are stonewalling ourselves, others or Heaven, we won't have to face the whip. We can change before our refusal to change leads to pain.

Where we have pain, let us look for what is underneath that has created the situation. We can meditate on our symptom a moment, but do not stay caught there. What are the underlying emotions? What are the underlying judgments and needs that have led to our having to be whipped, before it caught our attention? There are always signals that occur before an issue crescendos into a problem. If we are wise, we are always on the lookout for such signals. I do not mean being over-careful. This leads to roles, suffocation, and heaviness. Awareness and intuition witness, rather than deny, what is occurring to us in our everyday life. Denial and disregard of signs and signals lead to rude awakenings.

Let us commit to being the smart horse. Where there is pain, let us commit to find and heal the roots. Let us commit to learning the lesson before life has to resort to the whip to get our attention, and make us move forward.

Lesson 9 – All Pain is From the Past

That all present pain comes from past pain is an amazing principle which I learned over 30 years ago through my professional and personal experience. I then relearned it when reading A Course in Miracles. About fifteen years later, in my association with psychiatrist, Dr. Gwendolyn Brooks of Kona, Hawaii, we discussed this concept known in psychiatry as "transference". Again, this states that all present problems are transferred from the past onto present people and situations. Or, as Gwen put it about anything that wasn't happy, "It's all transference!"

By 1980, I had been able to help a number of people free themselves of physical symptoms and issues by helping them clear up their emotional and psychological issues. I had already learned the power of the mind to heal present problems by clearing the root in the past. This is what Gestalt therapy calls "unfinished business." All of our present problems are part of our life experience, and come from past issues. These began to show as personal problems or relationship issues and they typically originated in our families. Our family issues come from a combination of ancestral issues and soul issues, what our soul wants us to learn and heal in this life. Whether we believe in past lives, or think of soul issues as just the agenda that the soul has set for us, soul issues still represent major unconscious patterns that we have to heal or suffer accordingly. The patterns and issues are the same, no matter what you call them or what metaphor you use to heal them.

All of our physical and emotional pain comes from the past, a past we haven't gotten over. We somehow didn't use the past situation to free ourselves. We missed opportunities to heal ourselves, and others, through bonding, forgiveness, or bringing forth gifts within us to transform those past situations as they existed then. So, now we have to face these past conflicts as they are reflected in a present problem.

If you get to the root of a problem in the past and heal it there, it transforms the whole issue. Sometimes there are a couple of main roots, as I found when I worked with an 80-year-old woman with allergies. She declared at the beginning of the session, "I'm allergic to everything." We found two main roots causing her allergies. We cleared up a heartbreak she had when she was 21 years old, and an ancestral problem that had been passed through her family since the Civil War. When these past issues were healed, all of her allergies cleared up except for her cat allergy.

We can finally shift the past and heal the roots of an issue when we get over our fear of being gifted and powerful and are willing to turn to the next, better page in our lives and go forward. Courage is needed to heal ourselves. When we have it, then a new chapter begins in our life that is much better. It is then that the real roots of the problems become available. I have worked with people whose physical issues cleared up right away, and with others who have chronic or supposedly incurable physical illnesses that cleared up as we worked. I have also worked with at least one person with chronic issues, whose fear of embracing their purpose and destiny, kept the healing moving forward at a snail's pace. If you're willing to change significantly, you can clear up the past and move forward.

> If you are willing, ask how many root situations you need to clean up to heal the physical issue you are working with...

> If you were to know, how many began before, how many during and how many after your birth?

> If after your birth, it probably happened at the age of...

> If you were to know who was involved, it was probably you and...

> If you were to know what was going on, it was probably...

> If the incident was before your birth, ask yourself if it was in the womb or before that. It was probably...

> If it was in the womb, ask yourself what month it was...

> If it was before the womb, ask yourself if it was from the ancestral or soul level...

> If it is one of these, skip to the ancestral or soul level healing exercise below...

If in the womb ask what month it was...

Or if it was at birth, ask yourself: if you were to know who was involved, it was probably...

If you were to know what occurred, it was probably something like...

Now, let's go change your experience and help yourself and those in that incident to heal. Whatever the situation, imagine yourself back there before the trauma began.

Now, imagine the light within you connecting with the light inside everyone there.

Now, repeat this exercise of joining your light to theirs, but have their light come back to join your light. Repeat this bonding exercise again. Notice the difference in how the situation looks and feels each time you do it. Repeat this again until you reach a place of wild joy or pure light with everyone.

This is a bonding exercise that will restore, heal, and return you and the situation to an even better place than before the situation began. It will also heal the root of the issue and, thus, the whole issue itself. Continue the exercise with everyone's light passing to everyone until there is only joy or light in the scene. Examine the scene to see how everyone and the situation is doing as a result of each bonding.

If the problem began ancestrally, ask yourself, if you were to know if it was passed through your mother's, your father's, or both sides of the family. It was probably...

If you were to know if the problem began with a man or a woman, it was probably a...

If you were to know how many generations back it began, it was probably...

If somehow you were to know what took place, it was probably something like...

If you were to know what they were looking to learn by having this event take place, it was probably...

An easy way to learn a lesson is to bond. Let's get back to the original situation and have the light in your ancestor(s) join everyone around them. Repeat this bonding exercise from your ancestor(s) light to everyone around them and back again to themselves. Repeat this until the situation turns into a happy one. When this occurs, bring the energy of this situation down through the family until it is passed to you and your children, or grandchildren if you have any.

If the issue is a soul agenda or a past life story, it can also be healed with bonding...

In a past life story ask yourself: if you were to know, what country you were living in, it's the country that is now called...

If you were to know if you were a man or a woman, you were probably a...

If you were to know how long ago it was, it was probably...

If you were to know what happened that caused the problem, it was probably...

If you were to know what lesson you were seeking to learn by having that happen, it was probably...

Now, go back to when you were a small child in that life and repeat the bonding exercise with everyone and everything until there is only light and joy. Do this same exercise as you go through that life.

How does that life turn out now? Bring the bonded energy through that life and, bring it all the way through to your present life now.

If you believe the issue you are dealing with is a soul agenda, but you don't believe in past lives, ask yourself these questions:

If I were to know what key lesson I had set up for my life now regarding this issue, it is probably a lesson about...

If I were to know the gift I had come to give in this life to help myself and everyone, it was probably...

Now, go back to the time of your conception and bond your light to the light of your parents and sibling(s). Do this many times from your light to theirs and from theirs to each other's, and back to you.

Do this until the whole scene turns to happiness or pure light. Then imagine bringing out your soul gift and sharing it with everyone and everything since this life began. Then receive the gift that Heaven has for your family and share it with them.

This bonding exercise is just one way to help you heal the past, as it interferes with the present. We will examine other ways as we progress.

Lesson 10 – All Pain is Self-Attack

Trent had been rushed to the hospital with an acute asthma attack. When he got out, he called me for a session to find out what was going on. As we began to piece things together, we found a number of issues, including a fear of going forward to settle financial issues from the divorce with his ex-wife. Trent had been attacked so much in the relationship that he just did not want to deal with her any more. I pointed out to him that his wife's attack on him reflected his level of self-attack. Even though Trent had gotten out of the attack situation that came from being with her every day, he was now attacking himself for his refusal to deal with her. Even as we talked, he began a litany of complaints about his ex-wife for making his life so difficult, and then against God for doing the same thing.

God is the Prime Principle of Love. As such, He could never give us a hard life, illness, a bad marriage, etc. So, if God isn't doing that to us, the only common element in all of our painful situations in life is us. This is exactly what I have found in the subconscious ever since I began working in it. Every setback, problem, or painful situation is just a form of us attacking ourselves. Then we blame others and, whether we recognize it or not, we blame God for what is happening to us. We cut off our awareness of grace and the solution God gives us for every problem. Meanwhile, we are busy framing others and using them as an instrument in our self-attack.

Trent had a Self-Attack Conspiracy that he was using to hide the mastery level gift of Valuing - valuing himself and others, and knowing how much God valued him. As he realized this gift of Valuing, it gave him a great deal of relief and "breathing room."

I have found the dynamic of self-attack to be a part of every illness and painful situation. Everything negative that ever happened to us has an element of self-attack in it. If I look back over my work of almost four decades in the healing profession, I'd have to say that self-attack with its myriad of disguises is the number one problem in the world.

Attack from others is one of the toughest elements we have to face in life, but it would not faze us if we weren't also attacking ourselves. If we weren't attacking ourselves, we would recognize the attack of others on us as a call for help, and it would call forth our compassion. It is important for us to be compassionate to ourselves. Without it there is no true compassion for others, only sacrifice masquerading as sympathy.

Today, categorically commit to give up self-attack. Ask God's help for this on an ongoing basis. Anytime you catch yourself in self-attack, whether from the inside or disguised as an outward attack, use the simple healing method of helping another. Every self-attack comes from a personality, one of our many self-concepts. It is there to keep us from realizing that someone is in even greater need than we are. When in pain or other forms of self-attack ask yourself, "Who needs my help?" Then respond with love through the self-attack. This will pop you both into a flow. If you lose the flow because another layer of self-attack comes up, simply repeat the exercise. Do this until you are happy and in a continuous flow. Use it whenever you recognize you are not in the flow.

There is no self-attack posing as a problem that won't respond when we answer the calls for help around us. Every time you respond to calls from those who need your help, the problem, or a layer of it, is removed and you are brought into greater flow. It is the leadership principle: you make others more important than your self-attack. The steps in this are simple. First, become aware that you are attacking yourself. Second, ask who needs your help. Third, respond to them with love. If there is anything else to do or to say, you will be inspired with it. Enjoy the flow and recognize whether you have collapsed the problem or simply healed a layer of it. If it is only a layer, repeat the exercise until it is complete. Your responsiveness to the needs of others is one of the great healing principles. I have seen it work on the deepest layers of pain and remove layer after layer of chronic problems.

Lesson 11 – What You Think of Yourself

To be ill, to be in pain, we must think terrible things about ourselves. When we think such things about ourselves, they become terrible beliefs. As a result we hate what we believe about ourselves, and we want to attack ourselves. We can't will to destroy ourselves but we can will to destroy what we believe we are. While this can all be subconscious, it is no less destructive. We seek to destroy the image we have made of ourselves, but we cannot destroy our spirit. It is how we were created by God, and it can't be changed. We cannot destroy our soul-mind. It is the essence of us in time, though it can be filled with dark beliefs and self-images. We can displace these onto our body, and suffer as a result.

Isn't it time to discover these dark beliefs and self-images and let them go in the name of truth? Only what God believes about us can be true, and He can only think of His children as He thinks of Himself. The rest is a dark story we have made in which we are the villain. This cannot be true. It's not how God wills it, and it is not how we want it in our true will. Our ego revels in dark glamour even at the expense of our body.

Choose again! Give up seeing yourself as victim and as judge. Give up any dark or weak notions you have of yourself.

Lesson 12 – All Pain is Self-Punishment

Our ego is devious. We wouldn't stand for whipping ourselves or beating ourselves up. We accomplish our self-punishment in much more insidious ways. We get others to attack us. We suffer accidents or mishaps in life. We are "victims" of illness. Yet, in the subconscious mind, there is no such thing as an accident. Illness must have our name signed on the contract before it is delivered. All of this has guilt as one of its dynamics. When we have guilt, we punish ourselves in an attempt to alleviate or exonerate the guilt.

Self-punishment to alleviate guilt is obviously an ego strategy, because it is characteristic of all ego strategies in that they don't work. They always create more and bigger problems. Also, when the ego helps us with a problem, the trail to the root of the problem becomes obfuscated and confused. Punishment momentarily alleviates, then increases and reinforces the guilt. It is obviously the wrong direction.

If you are suffering in any way, ask yourself what you are punishing yourself for, what is it you feel you did wrong or didn't do right.

Guilt builds the ego, and the self-punishment that comes from the guilt darkly glamorizes it. You could correct the mistake instead with Heaven's help. What do you want: self-punishment or the solution of your higher mind? If you choose your higher mind, let your guilt and self-punishment go because it is a mistake. If you need some motivation, reflect on this: if you choose self-punishment, you will to the same extent punish or allow punishment on those you love.

Relax and open your mind. See what your higher mind suggests instead.

Lesson 13 – Self-Punishment for Family Guilt

Our family pattern is the primordial pattern of our lives. It is made up of unconscious patterns from ancestral and soul levels of the mind. Unless we, as well as our family, are operating at a mastery level of consciousness, we still have family guilt and most of it is subconscious. Underneath all of the family problems, failures, and grievances, we have levels of failure and guilt, compensated by roles, sacrifice or self-punishment in an attempt to make up for the guilt. This affects our relationships to the extent that we are either a victim, remain somewhat independent, or carry many burdens in order to make up for the caches of family guilt for which we are forever punishing ourselves.

I spent close to four decades researching the complicated patterns of the subconscious mind, made up of family and relationship patterns of heartbreak, guilt, failure, and compensation. There is a prodigious amount of guilt to pull up from the depths of our mind, guilt that our ego has convicted us of and that we have believed and therefore invested in with regard to our family. Our best option is to commit to healing our relationships and our family patterns. If we carry any issue from the past, it has now become a vicious circle of traps and guilt. Even if we were the one victimized, we carry guilt from those events.

What's fair about that? Nothing!

Guilt never pretended to be fair or true. It just promised that we should feel bad. It was our fault, and we should punish ourselves accordingly, or hide our guilt through dissociation. This made it less accessible, and all the while we blamed others for the guilt and failure we mistakenly bought into. It is our guilt that fuels judgment, grievances and our desire to punish. Those old traumas in our lives, where we were victimized, were always, at one level, an attempt to pay off family guilt.

The surface level of guilt is the level in which we felt we did something wrong or failed to do something right. The next level of guilt is the guilt we carry subconsciously. This contains all our family dynamics, such as causing a family member to lose because of our competition, sexual and aggressive feelings and thoughts, and, in general failing to save our family.

Guilt is made to keep us stuck but, where we give ourself fully as we do when we commit, we cut through the illusion of it and correct the mistake it was based on. Commit to the truth. Commit to healing, commit to bonded relationships and families. Giving oneself fully, as well as forgiveness, is an easy way to get past our hidden guilt.

If you do not forgive family members and yourself, you will pass on your hidden guilt to everyone you love and you will stay withdrawn, even if they need you. So many times pain or illness is a form of the martyr or needy role in the family. It is rare for these roles actually to help the family because roles are a form of co-dependency. Helping our family is much better accomplished through love, success, forgiveness and generosity.

Your pain or health problem now is tied in with old, untrue family guilt. Correct these mistakes, learn your lessons, help your families - but don't carry your family on your back because that is using them to hold yourself back. Forgive yourself and others or you will repeat the problems of the past, punishing yourself on the inside and out.

Families are meant to be support systems, not guilt generating mechanisms for life. Each of your family members shows you major soul patterns to heal in this life, so forgiveness will free you all. Also commit to your family members because no one gets better without help. Watch out for any tendency to fall into fusion or sacrifice. Use the 'sword of truth' to cut the attachment cords, so bonding will spring up in the place of attachments. As there are so many layers of attachment, co-dependency and sacrifice, it may take many cuts to realize a bonded relationship. Attachment is an attempt to get another to fill our needs and this is counterfeit love. Attachment always leads to pain. So let your attachments go so there can be the ease and freedom that comes of partnership and bonding. This will replace family guilt with empowerment and success.

Lesson 14 – Misuse of the Body

There are three main ways to misuse the body. If we use the body for pride, pleasure, or attack, we put our bodies at risk.

The ego makes us think we are our bodies, rather than that we are using the body as a vehicle for communication and learning. If used truly, the body is virtually inexhaustible. The extent to which we feel pride for our bodies separates us from others by putting us above them, and attempting to make us more deserving of special attention. To the extent we inflate ourselves about our body, we will also later knock ourselves down. Sooner or later the ego rejects the body as not being good enough for it. It tries to get rid of the body, sometimes with lethal results.

Twenty-five hundred years ago the Buddha recognized that if we sought pleasure we would find pain to the same extent. When we seek anything other than the peace of God we can easily split our mind in such a way as to create vicious circles of pain-pleasure, or pride-self torture. Pleasure is natural and comes to us from living naturally. But to seek pleasure, the second misuse of the body, is to be addicted to it or to make it an idol and this puts us in jeopardy.

When we use the body for domination through attack, withdrawal or keeping another in thrall to us, we do the very same thing to ourselves as we are doing to others. When we have misused the body, we pay for it in the coin of physical or emotional pain. It is important to put our body under the guidance of our higher mind rather than under our ego. Our higher mind will use the body for learning, sharing and as an indicator of what needs healing.

You could choose to do that right now. You could choose to do that everyday. You could reflect on which of these three ways you might be mis using your body. When did you make the decision to do this? Imagine yourself back at that juncture, but this time turn your mind and body over to your higher mind to direct. You have evidence of what happens when you chose to misuse your body under your ego's guidance. You can make a choice for the truth now. Back at that juncture, choose to center yourself simply by asking your higher mind to do so. Notice any difference in yourself and the situation. Now, ask again to be carried to your center and notice the difference. Do this until the situation has become one of love and happiness and you will naturally use your body for integrity.

Lesson 15 – The Chronic Resistance of Chronic Illness

A chronic illness or injury both conceals and reveals. An experience like this is, typically, so consuming that it distracts us away from the real issue at hand. In a chronic problem there is some deep seated conflict, and there may be many small conflicts in the way even before we become aware of the big one. A chronic illness shows that there is something we are resisting, but it occurs in such a way that we do not appear resistant. This resistance can be something major that happened a year or two before the onset of the illness; it could also be something that has just happened, is about to happen, or it may be a lifelong issue. We can use our health problems to reveal what was hidden away, by using the illness as an indicator of some area in our lives which is not working and that needs healing. We can use our resistance to see where the conflict lies.

Resistance and pain always go together. First, an illness begins with emotional pain, which builds up and is dissociated until finally it is too big to dissociate and is displaced to the physical level. Whenever the pain and resistance began, it speaks of an unlearned lesson and a time when we built up our egos at the expense of our lives.

Resistance that is more recent, speaks of a newly emergent issue that has not been accepted or integrated. Resistance from childhood reflects a place of soul level resistance that shows up as a family pattern. This is usually a lesson we are asked to learn, one that we judged and cannot abide in regard to our family. We may seem to have gone along with the program, but secretly we resisted and rebelled. Sooner or later, this can turn into an illness. Where we are in conflict, we do not move forward and consequently some vital flow in our lives is blocked. Eventually, this affects our health.

Our resistance may show as some kind of fight with authority or it may be turned against those we are in a work or love relationship with.

An illness is a fight without seeming to fight. An injury is a judgment without seeming to judge. We may act correctly, but the resistance and authority conflict eat away at us until there is some kind of health issue. The fact that there is a chronic illness speaks of the fact that there is a chronic issue which we have felt unable to face and resolve.

One of the great healing principles is simply to witness the issue. As we witness, we first become aware and then naturally accept that we are resisting, what we are resisting, and why. We simply give attention to what we are doing without judgment. What we accept is naturally let go of, and we move into a flow where we were stopped. The ego dissolves in this place, and there is more connection to our self and others.

Today take some time to reflect on any chronic illness or injury. If you have none, you can choose some niggling symptom.

- What is it you are resisting? Reflect on that.
- What is it that you are rebelling against? Reflect on that.
- What is the emotion you do not want to deal with?
- Witness what it is that you are fighting against without seeming to fight.

In a conflict you feel you cannot accept both sides at the same time. Do not judge either side. You believe you are the rebel, and what you rebel against. Now, take the rebel and what you rebel against, and instead simply witness them until both sides begin to change, meld together, and generate a flow. This place, which has been a monument to your ego, can be turned into a monument of healing and confidence.

Lesson 16 – Help From Above

Heaven is trying to help you in every moment and in every circumstance. Especially when you are hurting, know that Heaven is attempting to get through the fog of pain to help you. Whatever your path in life, Heaven wants to help you now. You do not need a spiritual path to ask for the Love that is *All That Is* to help you. And It will.

Sit quietly. Do not ask for help with your symptoms, but ask for love to heal the fear that is generating these symptoms. There can be no pain if there is no fear. It is fear that leads to the pain. Fear is a form of resistance. It separates us from ourselves, others and God. When it becomes strong, there is dissociation. When it builds up, the emotional pain becomes hidden, turning into a physical symptom that includes physical pain.

Now, sit with the fear that led to your pain. Let it surround you and ask that the fear, which is an illusion, be replaced with love, which is the truth. Let all your fear be released in this way. "Ask and it shall be given to you," was something Jesus said. Today, let grace, which is God's Love for you, be yours.

This is actually why healing can occur. Fear which creates the symptoms is an illusion. Love is the truth and as love and truth come into the picture they dissolve fear, bringing freedom and bonding instead of pain and bondage.

Lesson 17 – I am Under No Laws, But God's

This is one of my favorite lessons from *A Course in Miracles*.

It is another spiritual lesson to help us realize that in truth, the laws of the world are not God's laws. The laws of the world have built up over eons. They are part of our consensual reality, and, as such, they have the force of our mind behind them, generating the world we live in. The laws of the world are there to support our egos. Yet, we do not have to be bound by these laws. We may have bought into the laws of the world tens of thousands of times, yet this can all be reversed by a sincere change of heart. We cannot set our mind in the direction of the world and toward timelessness at the same time. We will be pointed in one direction or the other. Eventually our soul will make the right choice and evolve toward seeing the world with greater spiritual vision. This will free us of many of the traps we have gotten ourselves into.

"I am under no laws, but God's," is a declaration of freedom. I am not bound by the laws of the ego. My recommitment to my spiritual heritage gives me back my freedom. I do not have to suffer in any way because "I am under no laws, but God's." This is the beginning of embracing myself as spirit. Let us call on Heaven's help to release our investment in the ego. Then, we can choose to recognize God's laws as the only ones that bind us. This returns us to the power that is available to us when we realize we are spirit.

Lesson 18 – None Should Suffer

It is not God's will that we suffer. God could not remain God and wish such things on his children. Even if, at the level of spirit, our bodies and our sufferings are illusions, still God would not wish that we or anyone else experience suffering. This is so, even while we believe we are bodies in a world of time. In spite of our experience of the world and time - the result of our illusory experience of separation, it would still be mean to wish suffering on us in our believed helplessness. God is still God, and Christ is still the Christ. God is Love, and Christ His Awakened Son. Mary is still the mother of the Christ. Buddha is the Buddha. Quan Yin is still the Goddess of Mercy. Muhammed is still the prophet. All they could wish for us is the very best. Here is a quote from the Christ in *A Course in Miracles*, "I will, with God Himself, that none of His Sons should suffer."

No one in Heaven wants us to suffer. In our true will, we do not want to suffer. Today, let us receive all the love and grace of Heaven. Let us release our mistaken ego-agendas. Let us claim all the goodwill and support that is available to us. Our will, which is our spirit, is aligned with the Will of God. Let us align our heart, mind, and soul with our spirit. Let us reawaken to ourselves. Let us invoke Heaven's power. Let us know ourselves as we really are. Let us be healed because it is God's will that none should suffer.

Lesson 19 – Reconnecting

When we experience ourselves as sick, we experience ourselves as in need. This means we are experiencing ourselves in lack. Yet, at a subconscious level, we can only be deprived of something if we stop valuing it. This means that we valued something more than what or whom we lost. Many times, this occurred in childhood when we were making decisions to be independent or to have things our own way. We had victim experiences and we gave up some of our relatedness with our parents, so that we could have this independence, but it never made us happy. Every time we accepted an offer from the ego, it eventually led to fear and feelings of deprivation as a result of separation, which the ego is made of. There is no problem that does not have separation at its root.

Today, imagine yourself in the Hands of God, reconnected to all of your dear ones. Tonight when you go to sleep, sleep in God's arms. Do this reconnection every day and every night.

Lesson 20 – All Pain Comes From Attachment

Twenty-five hundred years ago the Buddha said that all pain comes from attachment. This could be said of physical pain as well as emotional pain. Where there is attachment, there is resistance as a defense. But sooner or later there is loss, so we have set up a vicious circle between attachment, loss and fear. Attachment is one of the defenses that comes from loss. We attempt to make up for our loss by holding onto something or someone to get the need met that the lost bonding had provided.

Imagine that all of your physical or emotional pain was actually a loud complaint about losses that you have experienced. Take something that hurts and reflect on what was so rudely taken away from you, not just as a result of the physical problem, but what loss you experienced beforehand that led to what is causing your pain now.

If you can accept your losses, you can move on from them. If you resist your losses, you will get stuck in emotional or physical pain. These are complaints that really hurt. If you let go and trust, something better will come to take the place of your loss. There will be a greater bonding and more happiness.

Repeat this exercise as many times as is necessary to let go of the losses that are causing your present pain.

Examine the pain you are in now, or a significant painful event from the past. Ask yourself:

If I were to know how many losses I am trying to make up for with my attachment(s) that led to the pain, it's probably

If I were to know how old I was when the loss occurred, it was probably

If I were to know who was involved, it was probably

And what occurred that brought about the loss was probably something like

Now, imagine that all those who love you are surrounding you, including all your friends in High Places. With all their love, feel your way through each loss. Remember, there may be other feelings or losses after this first one burns away. Go down through every level until all you are feeling is the love that surrounds you. This love will rebond you, healing the loss and pain that is the complaint.

Lesson 21 – Projection, Anger and Assault

All of us project. It is how the world was made. We took what we judged and rejected about ourselves, and we repressed it. But, because we could not stand the guilt of what we hated about ourselves and which was split off and buried, we projected it out on the world. What we see in the world is what we have judged about ourselves. We simply don't like, and feel threatened by, these parts of ourselves. That is why *A Course in Miracles* states that our purpose is to forgive the world. What we see in the world is what we have judged about ourselves and are, thus, afraid of. Love, forgiveness, understanding, and all other forms of bonding, draw us together and win back peace and wholeness for us.

Our perception shows us our self-concepts. Thus, when we are angry at someone, they reflect a belief we have about ourselves. We can only be angry at ourselves. Our shadows, based on guilt, eat away at us with hidden self-hatred. When we get angry at someone, we are attacking ourselves once again and any self-attack weakens us. When we attack others, or when others attack us, we have subconsciously set up the situation in an attempt to ameliorate our guilt. This, of course, never works. It only succeeds in making us feel worse, which simply brings more guilt, more self-punishment and attack, in a vicious circle.

Our projections are a defense that the ego has promised will help us, but they actually hide the problem and make us less available for healing what needs to be healed. If we project on others, in itself a form of anger, judgment, and attack, and then attack them directly, we reinforce our own self-hatred. This is very bad for our health. A projection means an intrapsychic conflict has also become an interpersonal conflict with someone in our world. Anger and attack on anyone is an attack on ourselves first. This is also bad for our health. We cannot attack another without attacking ourselves. Even to be in the vicinity of one person attacking another shows our inner conflict, one part of us attacking another part of ourselves.

Look out at your world. Who out there deserves to be attacked and tortured? Notice where you are similarly attacking and torturing yourself. How is this affecting your health?

If you have pain, it is not just a matter of attacking yourself. Self-attack cannot be simply focused on yourself. If you attack yourself, you are attacking others around you, including those closest to you. I once worked with a European whose hatred of President Bush was so virulent that it turned out to be at the root of her cancer. She had come for a coaching session on the day the doctors had predicted she would die because she was so cancer ridden. On this day, besides healing her hatred of President Bush, she also healed her hatred toward her ex-husband, and the devastating guilt she felt in regard to her mother. While this session dealt with only the tip of the iceberg, she lived another year and a half as a result. Her anger at President Bush and her ex-husband, as well as her guilt, all had earlier roots. Her anger and self-anger stemmed back to significant relationships from her past, with both childhood and unconscious roots.

You can use your anger as an indicator of conflict within yourself, which shows you what needs healing, or you can use it as a justification to assault another. One will greatly increase your pain, though your attack will momentarily distract you from the pain of your self-attack.

You can use anger as an indicator that you are making a mistake, because anger is impossible without projection, and choose healing. On the other hand you can build your righteous attack, further wounding yourself.

Reflect on your biggest experience of being angry and judging someone. What was going on? Who was it with?

If this incident was trying to let you know of an earlier conflict, it happened at the age of

It involved you and

The conflict you are dealing with from before was about

If you forgive this original person and yourself, it will be much easier to forgive the person you are angry at or judging now.

One way to forgive is to join your mind with God and to see this person as a part of you, just as you are part of God. As judgment dissolves, so does the separation, and as separation in your mind and toward others dissolves, so does your pain.

Lesson 22 – Letting the Holy Spirit

To experience ourselves as sick is to experience ourselves as outside the Kingdom of God, Heaven and the awareness of Oneness, of which we are all a part. We are both a creative thought extending from the Mind of God and an act of love extending from Love. We are enfolded in the Mind of God, still in His Love. The belief that we are not, is the notion of separation on which the ego founds itself - that what was One could be separated.

> "Sickness and separation are not of God...to heal, then is to correct perception in your brothers and yourself by SHARING THE HOLY SPIRIT WITH HIM. This places you both WITHIN the Kingdom, and restores ITS wholeness in your minds."

A Course in Miracles original text

The Holy Spirit is the connection between us and God, and between us and all others. It is the Remembrance of the relatedness of all things. As we share this Remembrance, we remember ourselves. We allow perception and history to fall away, and we experience that we are joined with all beings and with Being. How could there be loneliness or separation? How could we feel outside the Kingdom? Welcome the Holy Spirit, and share the Holy Spirit to let your pain and separation dissolve. You will remember what has been long forgotten and it will bring you peace and make you happy.

Lesson 23 – Aligning with God and Creation

To align with God and Creation is to become healed once again. God and all Creation are one, and this includes us. But we have made another will, other than God's. This is our ego's will and in the life it would give us it would make us both gloat and suffer. The ego is that part of us that wants our own way.

We fight God because we want to be God. We want separation. We have made a dream life apart from God's Will. God wants only love and happiness for us, but we have dreamed a world of suffering and death. In our self-deception, we rage against God as if He were the cause of our suffering. We have made endless dissociations, so that we have lost the Oneness of God and creation. We have lost the exquisite taste of Heaven and framed God for our leaving.

We cannot think we are a body and not suffer. We cannot have self-concepts and not suffer. Our beliefs wall us off from God and Creation. Yet, nothing has changed; we only dream it has. As we align our will with God's Will, we begin the awakening process. We remember our health and wholeness. Layer after layer of the chimera falls away, and the joy returns in a gentle awakening process. Our power returns because it was given to us by the All Powerful.

Wheel alignment in a car helps save the tires from extra wear and tear. It makes for a smooth ride. Similarly, alignment with God's Will cuts down the resistance and gives a smooth ride through life. As the dissociation falls away, we are more open to guidance and grace. All that we have buried will come to the surface to be easily released. The negative comes up and, as it is healed, the positive begins to grow exponentially. As we align with God, we begin to remember what was forgotten and what we remember is Love. We remember Heaven, the remembrance of Oneness as it is within us and has always been within us. As we remember this, we recognize it and know that we are unchanged from how we were created.

Today, align yourself with the Great Spirit of life, and you will remember how much you are loved and to know that, is to know love, health and alignment to truth.

Lesson 24 – The Mind is Most Open

The mind is most available to us without ego interference just before we fall asleep and just when we wake up. The ego agendas have fallen away or not yet re-engaged first thing in the morning, so this makes it the best time to use our mind to heal pain. As we learn how effective it is to use our mind at these times of the day we will, by the results of our work, naturally gravitate toward making use of this important time. Early and late in the day are the best times to set up what kind of day we want to have.

These night and morning times are the best to visualize your general health and well-being and specifically to work on any area of your body that needs special attention. You can visualize, feel, and sense that area of your body as vibrant, healthy, and whole.

You can use that time to love yourself and know yourself as innocent. You can manifest the kind of day you want: peaceful, energetic, and happy. You can sense specifically the things you want to have happen. If other things occur in your day that are negative, it shows ego agendas and subconscious patterns interfering. As these things occur, realize this is not what you want, and it was a mistake to choose it. Then choose again the kind of day you want and what you would like instead.

Actually, anytime of day can be used for inner healing when you take the time to use it on your behalf. For example, when traveling in a particularly bumpy, small plane to the Okanagan, British Columbia, I began to get nauseated. I manifested (vividly saw, felt, and sensed) that, in ten minutes, I would no longer feel sick. Ten minutes later I felt only a slight queasiness, so I began to work on manifesting for the flight itself to be smooth. Within ten minutes we had a smooth flight the rest of the way, whereas twenty minutes before it had been a tumultuous flight.

To manifest, you simply need to choose what is believable to you and to visualize, feel, or sense vividly what you would like to occur. Another way is to see, feel and sense what you want to have happen as *already done*.

Use your mind to help yourself. It is your greatest asset besides your heart and spirit. Positive thinking, for the most part, is a thin veneer of positive thought over an ocean of negativity. Whereas, using your mind to bring about the results you wish can begin the transformation of the ocean. Be your own best friend rather than your own worst enemy. Use your mind frequently to change your life for the better, especially in the early morning and late night.

Lesson 25 – The Incorrigibility of Pain

The body is the whipping boy of the mind. When we have a conflict that we cannot resolve, we displace it onto the body. In that sense, the body pays for the 'sins' of the mind. Where we believe we have sinned, where we believe we are guilty, we punish ourselves. Guilt keeps us stuck and demands self-retribution.

Pain shows a place where we are in conflict and are not moving forward. The holding on and refusal to progress, brings about the resistance that generates pain. In most cases, the conflict that brings about our pain is not even conscious, which is why the body becomes an easy dumping ground for our emotional issues.

Pain reflects a place of lost flow and blocked energy. It shows some conflict that we did not find the answer to, but tried to trudge on in spite of. As our conflicts accumulate, the body becomes an easy place for pain to congregate.

The greater our refusal to change, the greater the pain. The pain nags or even batters, distracting us, but we could use it as an indicator that there is something that we are adamantly refusing to let go of, and graduate from. The more serious the pain, the bigger the leap to the next chapter in our lives, which would be that much better. The area in which we are frozen is our ego's attempt to limit our healing. There is some issue we are afraid to face; there is an area that we are afraid to change. There is some step we just will not take. And though we are afraid of it, it is a step forward in our lives. It will bring us to a new and better way.

Let us take the example of the death of a beloved life partner. If we do not let our partner go, we ourselves begin heading in a death direction. In most cases, this is not the truth, and we are called to go on to the next stage in our lives where a better life awaits. If we let go partially, then our life is limited as we go on, but there is no renaissance in our lives. As a result, we do not fully experience all the love our partner, who has gone before, gave to us because we did not let them go. This does not honor our relationship with our partner who is deceased, nor does it honor what that partner would wish for us now. To let our partner go, allows for all the love they gave us to become part of us, and opens the way to the next, better chapter in our lives. This may possibly contain a new partner for our next stage. This is not a betrayal of our former partner; it was made possible by the love our former partner gave to us.

As we find that place in which we are unamenable to change; we find a place where we think we know best. We find a place where we want things to be "our way." This is not in our best interest, as it holds us back from the vicissitudes of the next step, which does not contain pain. We cannot possibly know what Heaven has in store for us, but it is certainly not pain or suffering or Heaven would lose its Heaven license. Heaven has a plan for us to be happy, if we would simply accept it and trust enough to go forward. It would allow the next stage to simply unfold in our lives. This would naturally include either the gradual or immediate disappearance of pain, or in our finding a new medical treatment that would succeed in easing the pain.

Your incorrigibility is a stubborn refusal to change to that which is in your best interest. Choose to become aware of what you have hidden from yourself and let that go. Be motivated to change. Be willing to change. Commit to the next stage in your life. Commit to yourself and what would really make you happy.

Lesson 26 – Do I Want the Problem or Do I Want the Answer?

This question is an important one to ask because, if we truly want the answer, we will find it. If we want the problem of pain, we will keep it in spite of all the help, doctors or medicines that come our way. The answer is as simple as the answer to this question: "Do I want the problem or the answer?" Heaven would not bid us suffer in any way. If a loving parent would not will their child to suffer, how could God will us to suffer?

When our children were babies, I once heard our pediatrician, who was also an oncologist, say, "I have known good, bad and indifferent parents, but there is not one of those parents who would not take the place of their child when that child is suffering." God could not wish suffering on anyone and remain the principle of Love. If it is not Heaven who bids us suffer, then there is only one left who would have us suffer. It's not pretty what we do to ourselves, nor is it true, but it is true that *we do it to ourselves*. This is helpful in that we are not helpless in the face of our pain. If it is we who have decreed that we suffer, then it is also we who can re-decide. To do this, we must eschew all guilt and take total responsibility for what is happening. We must want to find what we have hidden from ourselves and immediately turn it over to Heaven to be redone for us.

I have spent close to four decades wandering the hidden places of the ego. Here are some of the key reasons we make ourselves suffer.

Now, choose three numbers from one to twelve. Before you turn the page, check out which numbers you wrote down. They will reflect your dynamics in regard to the pain.

1. Idol of the Ego - to build our ego through suffering.
2. Idol of Martyrdom - the attempt to save someone through suffering. Who would that be? What led you to believe that your suffering would save them?
3. A Monument to a Loss You Suffered. Your pain is a signal of how much your loss meant to you, but your pain does not honor the person you lost only the greatness you accomplish would honor them.

4. A Heartbreak You Are Still Suffering, displaced onto the physical.
5. An Act of Revenge on someone. Who could this be?
6. The Idol of Guilt and Self-Punishment. You are wrongfully accusing and condemning yourself for a mistake that simply needs to be corrected.
7. The Idol of Self-Deprivation. You are worshiping the god of scarcity and robbing yourself of health and well-being. Peace is your legacy, which you have denied.
8. An Excuse to avoid your guidance and what you are called to do.
9. Holding on to Some Attachment or Indulgence that you believe you can have if you pay the price of pain.
10. Fear of Going Forward. You believe you are not up to the task of the next stage. No one could expect you to go forward, because you are suffering.
11. Fear of Leadership. Those around you need you, but you would rather suffer than take the responsibility. Yet, many more will suffer if you do not take your place and do what you can do.
12. Your Authority Conflict With God. Obviously, God is a bad God if you suffer like you do. You would rather refuse His gifts and suffer than recognize yourself as a Child of God. Your ego wants God's job, since God has obviously done so badly with you and the world, His job must be up for grabs if you suffer.

These are a few of the core dynamics that you use against yourself in your pain. But you can stop investing in pain and in your underlying dynamics. Heaven has a better plan, if you acknowledge your mistakes and ask for help. Let go of your dynamics and choose a better way. Let Heaven show you and do it for you.

Heaven wants you happy and free. It is time to give up your investment in hell. It's certainly no place for vacation.

Lesson 27 –No Past, No Pain

If we had no past, we would have no pain. It is the unfinished business of the past that erupts causing us pain now. If not dealt with, emotional pain, conflict and guilt become displaced and carried in the body. We are poisoned by our judgments and the guilt underneath. All that is from the past. Shame lingers within us, limiting us by the self-concepts that it generates. Our positive and negative belief systems generate a conflicted world, while our negative belief systems have us perceive and experience the results of our self-attack. Whatever we believe about anything is actually a self-concept that comes from the past. These beliefs, even if positive, limit us while, if they are negative, they are both limiting and a cause for self-attack. Negativity breeds negativity and promulgates suffering. As we get older, this accumulates in the mind and, in our confusion, is pushed into the body leading to suffering. Our healing, especially as we forgive others and ourselves, lets go of attachment and grievances. This leads us to release the constantly accumulating debris of judgment, fostered by self-concepts.

If we lived only in the present, we would be centered and in peace. We would live in a world of pure goodness and grace, beyond the world of right and wrong and, therefore, beyond past generated self-concepts. We would also live a life where we would have let go of the past and its guilt, and not try to live in the future with its fear. When we live in the present, there is only peace – no sadness or regrets, and no concerns or worries. The more centered we are, the more we live in the present moment. This leads to peace and the more peaceful we become the more we realize a state of mastery, which naturally recognizes our value as a child of God. This leads to innocence, effectiveness and living with an identification of ourselves as beyond the body.

A Course in Miracles describes inner peace as healing. To get to peace, we must move beyond judgment, and to get beyond judgment, we must get beyond self-judgment. Only our forgiveness and self-forgiveness accomplishes this. Only our letting go of grievances and attachments will lead to the re-bonding necessary for peace and innocence.

Today, ask your higher mind to lead you back to your center and the peace that awaits you. Every few minutes, ask to be carried back to a progressively deeper and higher center. Do this throughout the whole day. Ask that anyone around you also be brought to a new center of peace.

When you are feeling the joy that comes from peace, choose the most painful experience in the last eighteen months. Ask to be centered in that event and notice how it feels and looks differently. Then ask to be brought to progressively higher and deeper centers until you pass beyond the pain of that situation to the sea of peace that brings joy. Notice how you feel and how the situation looks after each centering. Also, include anyone in that situation with you, and ask that they be brought to their center of peace. Next, choose the most painful event of your life and ask to be centered to the point of being utterly peaceful.

Repeat your centering exercises every day for a week. If you are totally dedicated, you could do it every day for the rest of your life, bringing profound peace and joy to yourself. This allows those past events to dissolve and brings you back to the present and success.

Lesson 28 – Pain as Authority Conflict

Pain is not only a message, a call for help to those around us, it also represents a conflict in our minds. At least part of this conflict reflects a fight, an attempt to defeat someone. This makes our pain an aspect of an authority conflict. Our pain is the victim part of a fight. Our pain is a finger of accusation, pointing to someone saying, "Look at what you did to me. It is because of you that I suffer". Naturally, we relegate these types of issues to the subconscious and unconscious mind as they are not fully acceptable to us.

All of our authority conflict could be traced back to our authority conflict with God. The fear within us gives away the hidden fight we have inside. What I have found, after three-and-a-half decades of work, is that any issue we have with anyone about anything, we also have with God.

In regard to your pain, ask yourself, "Who am I having a fight with? And what is it about?"

Next, ask yourself, "What am I blaming God for? What am I fighting with God about?"

Notice that God does not fight back. It is not within the nature of God to do so. God only gives; He does not take, in spite of our projections to the contrary.

God has already given us the answer to the present problem. It is the nature of God to do so. We are afraid to listen to God because we believe He will take from us and make us sacrifice. Again, this is not within God's nature, only within ours. Perfect Love only reaches out with perfect love and does not demand or take in any way. It is only our ego nature that does this. Then we project what we have done on God and those around us. This is the nature of guilt, judgment, anger and accusation. We have to project it, because we cannot stand what we mistakenly believe and feel about ourselves.

It is time to forgive ourselves for our anger and fights because they only come from our projection. Our anger is madness. It is killing us. It is time for us to eschew the ego and know ourselves as a child of God. Then we can listen to God's solutions for us because they will work if we adopt them. Maybe it's time to forgive those we have blamed, including

God, for mistakes we thought we made. Our forgiveness of others frees us both. Our forgiveness of God opens us to His miracles and frees us of pain.

Lesson 29 – Healing Back Pain

Pick a number between one and twenty-six. Write it down. If two numbers pop in to your mind, write them both down. The mind speaks in symbols, metaphors and puns. Thus, you can see the communication the mind makes by its different conflicts if you know how to read the body.

Back pain, especially involving the bones, speaks of soul or unconscious issues. The joints speak of issues of integration or joining, first with ourselves and then with others. It is the same for ligaments with more of an emphasis on our relatedness. What is in our body correlates with what is in our mind. Muscles have to do with our sense of strength or weakness. Overexertion on the outside speaks of the same thing on the inside in regard to how we are dealing with relationships (left side) and work (right side.) Hips reflect issues of change. The pelvis equals issues of flexibility, while the coccyx shows issues around fear, need, scarcity, loss, and resistance (the tail-between-the-legs syndrome, usually from childhood and soul level issues.) It can also reflect self-attack, especially about sex. Shoulders reflect burdens and trying to do things on our own rather than with others or with grace. The neck is about attitude, the connection between ideas, ideals and action. The head stands for thought and direction.

With all the metaphors there are to examine and play with, it is best to do so intuitively and lightly; analyzing defeats the purpose of re-establishing flow. All pain is meant to distract us and keep us from the flow. Analyzing makes everything heavy, which only serves the ego.

Issues of the back may also reflect the seven chakras going up the spine. Problems localized around these centers can have significance regarding that particular chakra:

The first chakra, in the coccyx, is about survival, vitality and sexuality.

The second chakra, three inches below the navel, represents self-worth and sexuality.

The third chakra, three inches above the navel, represents our power, success and self-expression.

The fourth chakra is the heart center but over the spine represents the heart and personal love issues.

The fifth chakra, in the neck, represents a second power center. It has to do with communication, leadership and impersonal love for everyone.

The third eye, or sixth chakra, in the forehead above and between your eyes, represents your thinking, creativity and vision center, connecting you with your purpose.

The crown chakra, on top center of your head, represents your opening to grace.

Again, it is important to use your intuitive sense around each energy center and their significance, to see if they have meaning for you. An old, tried and true way is to say a sentence out loud to see if it has the ring of truth. For example to say, "My lower back pain has to do with my feeling of unworthiness and sacrifice." To the extent this statement is true, it will feel and sound true to you.

Now, take the number you wrote down at the beginning and examine it in terms of the numbers below. The numbers below have been synchronistically correlated in regard to your back pain and its dynamics. If you become familiar with the numbers and what they signify, hereafter you may want to write the numbers on cards to pick from the pack to find your number in the future. Sometimes, there are a number of layers to be healed, especially around back pain.

Now take a look at what number popped up for you and what it means.

1. Resistance – You are "*backed-up*" about what is going on.
2. Sacrifice – You have saddled yourself with a big load.
3. Revenge – You are "getting *back*" at someone.
4. Betrayal – You feel "knifed in the *back*".
5. Withdrawal, Separation – You "*back away*" from life, others, yourself and the Divine.
6. Anger – You have your "*back up*".
7. Burnout – You're "breaking my *back*." Or the straw that broke the camel's back.
8. Holding-on – You are always looking *back*.

9. Victim – You feel "*back-ended*."
10. Greed, Need, Scarcity – "*Baksheesh*" – the Egyptian word for money. "Do you have baksheesh?"
11. Unsupported – You don't feel "*backed*" by those around you.
12. Fear – You are "*backing* down."
13. Rejection of something or someone – You are "*backing-off*."
14. Wounded – "Take *back* what you said and did; it hurt."
15. Sneaky, fear of bad surprises – If it does not get you through the front door, it gets you through the "*back door*."
16. Guilt over gifts, such as being luckier, more gifted or successful than other family members – "Holding oneself *back*."
17. The result of indulgence – "*Backanalia*" (Bacchanalia)
18. Dispossessing oneself, throwing oneself away, recklessness – "Throwing one's *back* out."
19. Lack of courage, will or moral fiber – "No *backbone*."
20. Desperate, cornered – "*Backed* into a corner."
21. Hitting back because of feelings of being wronged – "*Backlash*."
22. Fear of purpose and destiny. Lack of commitment – "*Backed out*."
23. Grievance – "*Backed up*."
24. Abandoned – "Lost your *backing*."
25. Stubborn, proud, adamant – "He won't *back* down."
26. Overwhelmed – "You're breaking my *back*."

Once you have found the issue, ask yourself if the issue feels old, ancient or primordial. Old represents childhood and family issues, while ancient relates to ancestral or soul patterns. Primordial represents the foundation, where we made the ego.

Mull over your issues for a while.

1. Then forgive yourself for displacing this issue into your body and for the issue itself. Forgive anyone else who was present when the issue began or as it compounded. Trust your intuition on this.
2. Give this over to Heaven. Once you have taken full responsibility for your back pain and its issue, turn it over to Heaven to undo it quickly for you.

In two days, notice how you feel, pick another number and repeat the exercise.

Lesson 30 – Giving Heals Pain

Anything that is blocked or conflicted within us leads to pain. Giving puts us back in the flow. Pain is a distraction from what needs to be healed. Giving focuses us on our relationship with those around us in a helpful way. Whether the pain is physical or emotional, giving can help. While some physical and emotional pain emerges from the very depths of our mind, our continuous giving can clear it, layer after layer, and help hold the pain at bay while the roots are healed.

What are some of the ways that we can give? We can give prayers, blessings, money, time, help, forgiveness, gifts, love, and friendship. You could ask intuitively who needs your help and you could imagine that your pain separated you from whoever comes to mind. Now, through your pain, give the love, blessings and gifts that they seem to need until it reaches them. If this does not take away the pain, repeat the exercise with whoever comes to your mind next. Sometimes, there are many layers of giving that need to be done. Sometimes, the nature of the pain is such that being in service only keeps the pain at bay. We may need to give significant gifts from within to help others, while at the same time dissolving our pain. These could include love, trust, happiness, abundance, friendship or thousands of other things that might come to mind. These gifts are all inside you. If you don't recognize a specific gift that the person who pops into your mind needs, then open one of the doors in your mind that seems to beckon you. Behind the door will be the gift that person needs. Embrace and share it. Also, you can receive from Heaven a gift they need and that Heaven wants to give them through you. The only cost for you to give it is, that you receive it also. Share this gift with the person who is in greater need than you. While at times you are called to give a physical gift or go to a person in need, most of the time you can simply do these exercises from mind to mind. Letting go of judgments can be especially good for you and others. They need help and you are giving it, thus availing yourself of the help you need. Giving heals pain.

Lesson 31 – Loving Yourself

All illness comes from lack of self-love. Pain is a step beyond this in that it is a form of direct self-attack. Pain comes from a conflict within that has become so acute that we are now punishing ourselves as a result. This is where loving ourselves is a healing balm to soothe the pain. Loving ourselves has been what is missing. It ends separation and division, which are the roots of illness. Separation and division with another begin with separation and division within ourselves. This all falls away as we realize the importance of self-love. Start now. Self-love rebonds us both with ourselves, others and Heaven.

Take some time to extend to yourself.

How could you give more to yourself?

What is in the way of loving yourself?

Choose to let that go.

Find the attachment that is causing the pain and let that go; it brings you only harm. Reach out to yourself. Bless yourself. Loving yourself re-bonds you, integrating some of the separation in your own mind and ending some of the conflict. This can ease your pain.

Spend five minutes loving yourself now. If this seems difficult, ask for Heaven's help to accomplish this. Then give five minutes to yourself.

Now go back to a time in your life when you were in a lot of pain, heartbreak or misery. Love yourself for five to ten minutes or as long as it takes for you to feel at peace back there.

Every hour, on the hour, for the next week, spend a minute loving yourself. You can simply take a moment if you are busy and need your full attention elsewhere. But many times you can carry on with what you are doing and still consciously love yourself.

Lesson 32 – To Love Yourself

Illness and injury reflect a place where we do not love ourselves. Similarly, pain reflects a place where we are not only not loving ourselves, we are actively attacking ourselves. What is it that you feel you deserve to be attacked for? Whatever it is, it is not the truth. You punish yourself and are caught in a Self-Attack Conspiracy, possibly an Illness Conspiracy. These are meant to keep you from your gifts and your purpose. They signal that you have followed the ego's agenda and the ego, based on deception, has no love for you.

Now, it is time to reverse that. You can heal yourself if you love yourself. There were so many times in your life that you threw yourself away. Through self-love, you can gain yourself back and have the substance to love others. Otherwise, when you start to love another, it is easy to fall into sacrifice instead of the true giving that comes of love. To love yourself, simply open your heart and give to yourself.

Today, choose the ten worst times of your life. Imagine yourself back there. Love yourself. Commit to yourself. Welcome back any part of you lost at that time. Love yourself until all judgments on yourself fall away. Love yourself until the love extends to everyone in that situation, and they can love themselves. Love yourself until even the roots that led to such a situation, melt away. To love yourself in that situation adds to the self-love in your situation now. It opens channels of love to you from yourself, others and the Divine.

Next, choose the second of your ten worst situations. Again, choose and commit to yourself. Be true to yourself and love yourself. Welcome any lost selves back. As in the first situation, love yourself until it extends self-love to all, and even melts away the roots that led to such a situation.

Next, go through the other eight worst times of your life, loving yourself and doing the same in every situation.

Lastly, give love to yourself now in the same way, until you can feel the joy of self-love in your life.

Lesson 33 – The Pain of Getting Older

Ahh! The many aches and pains of getting older. It's a natural thing, isn't it? We get older, and things wear out. That's the reality, isn't it? But maybe, just maybe, there is an alternative, one that is not only natural but supernatural.

It is in our nature to move beyond limitations. This is occurring as human consciousness evolves; this is occurring without us having to do anything. But, personally, we cannot wait thousands of years for that evolution to happen. We may have the aches and pains of aging going on already. We need a change for the better now.

So let us deal with it in the present moment.

(i) First, you may want to divest yourself of any personal belief systems you have about aging. Then let go of any belief systems about aging you may have picked up from the collective consciousness of consensual reality. Simply let them go; stop investing in them. Alternatively, put them in God's hands. He doesn't believe in them either. He doesn't believe in any limitation. Be on His team.

(ii) Next, begin manifesting for yourself, especially before you go to sleep at night and when you wake up in the morning. Visualize, feel, sense, and hear that you are feeling youthful, vibrant, and energized for the next day. Choose a happy day, a breakthrough, an easy, graceful, healthy day. See and feel this as vividly as possible. Want it with all of your heart! Give yourself five minutes at night and in the morning. Ask for a graceful day. Ask for the gift of rejuvenation. In truth, Heaven wills this for you. Will it for yourself. Will it for your partner or a parent who is suffering the effects of aging or illness. As you give to others in this way, you also give to yourself.

(iii) Ask yourself intuitively: "Who could I forgive that would help my health?" Whoever comes to mind, imagine them standing in front of you. Imagine someone you want to help standing next to them. Look past the body and personality of the one you want to help. Imagine you see the light within you joining with the light inside them. Now see the person you need to forgive. Look past their body and personality to the light inside them. Imagine the light of you and your friend now joining this person to become one light.

(iv) Imagine you were floating back through time and space to an incident that is at the root of your pain and which is now accelerating your aging process. Ask yourself:

If you were to know, how old were you?

If you were to know, who was present when this occurred?

If you were to know, what happened at this time?

If you were to know, what did you decide then that is affecting you negatively now?

If you were to know, what lesson were you looking to learn instead of the negativity you took on?

What is the gift from Heaven you are being given to assist you in healing or transforming that situation in a positive way?

Receive this gift along with any grace coming to you back there. Then share this gift with anyone who was in that situation with you. If this does not completely ameliorate the situation, then another gift awaits your pleasure. Receive that and share it also until everyone in that event is feeling great.

Lesson 34 – Loving the Part that Hurts

It is proven that we can change the chemistry of our bodies by our thoughts. For instance, we can send blood rushing to certain muscles if we imagine ourselves in action.

Love is the most positive of our feelings, and it can have the strongest effect to bring relief from pain and even to effect healing. If your pain reflects a place where you are attacking yourself, then it would make sense to love yourself instead of attacking yourself.

This next exercise is very simple. Everyday for the next month, put aside five minutes in the morning and five minutes in the evening for this exercise. You can also do this any time of the day or night that you wish, if only for a few seconds. Focus on the part of the body that is giving you the most trouble. Love it. Be grateful for it. Recognize what it has given you in your life. Warm up to it. Make friends with it. Listen to it. Encourage it. It has a message; it is in distress. Give to it. Wash it with love. Tell it you love it. Feel your heart gushing love like a spring for this part of you. Make this a meditation for yourself. As you give to your body, the conflict that led to the pain may begin to surface. Love yourself through the pain.

At times, when people first start this exercise, they report emotions coming up, such as self-hatred, self-loathing or sadness. Sometimes only resistance comes up. Do not judge or run from these feelings. They are actually very helpful because they are part of what's causing your pain. Love these aspects. Love the part of you that is loathing or judging you. Love it until it melts away. Then go on to spend whatever time is left loving the part itself.

If you are working on your weight or tiredness, it may affect your whole body. So simply love your whole body. In the evening, ask yourself how old is the self inside you that is suffering. Coach that self. Appreciate it. Love that self until it gets to your present age and melts back into wholeness within you. Sometimes people report loving some entity within them that seems entirely alien. It will leave you, going where it belongs if you love it enough.

Love the part of you that hurts. It reflects a part of you physically and mentally that needs help. Give that help. Ask Heaven to give its love for you through the love you give to yourself.

Lesson 35 – Waking From the Dream

A Course in Miracles speaks of our life as a dream. This coincides with the Buddhist belief about the world. I have found this concept to be true and practical in healing everyday situations. In the 1970's, I reveled in learning and developing techniques for transforming dreams as the gateway to the subconscious and unconscious mind. Then in the early 1980's, I realized that life was a dream also, and as such, all the dream methods could be applied to our daily lives with good effect.

Dreams are wish fulfillment. We need only examine a night of our dreams to see how chaotic and conflicting our wishes are. Wishes come from need or curiosity, but the effect is the same. They generate the waking and sleeping dreams of our lives.

In *A Course in Miracles*, it states that the original separation from Oneness began out of curiosity. Someone asked, "I wonder what it would be like to be separate." And everyone forgot to laugh at such a joke. As a result, we dreamed a world of separation. As far as I can tell by working deep in the mind, the original split is a place of terrible pain and meaninglessness – a place where we lost sight of our value. It is the birth place of the ego and this root is still inside our mind. This was the original "dark night of the soul." Then instead of simply waking up to Oneness out of willingness and desire, we began to dissociate the pain and we fled deeper into the dream. As we went deeper into the dream of this world, making it out of judgment, we became more and more split and experienced ourselves as both more separate and more asleep. Now we are returning to Oneness through a series of re-awakenings. Each awakening we have leads to an experience of greater love and unity.

It is so easy to believe in our waking life that the dream is real, especially when we are suffering. It is then that it is most important to remember that we are dreaming. And just as easily as when we release our night time dreams as unreal when we awake, we can do the same with our waking dreams and awaken to a more perfect world and eventually to Oneness.

As we learn what motivated us to dream a dream of suffering, it can be helpful for us to let it go. Ask yourself these questions and trust the answers that come to you.

What this dream of pain allows me to do is

What this dream of pain gives me the excuse not to do is

The indulgence I get to keep in this painful dream is

(Especially be aware of emotional and authority conflict types of indulgence.)

How this dream of suffering helps me avoid my purpose is by

The gift I'm especially avoiding by staying in this bad dream is

The reason I'm avoiding this gift is because I

What I am trying to get or achieve by this painful dream is

The person I am getting revenge on by having this dream of pain is

The dream of guilt I am trying to pay off with my dream of pain is

The attachment I am holding onto through this dream of pain is

Once you see some of the motivation behind your dream of pain, you might be motivated to let the dream go as a bad deal.

It will help if you want to be awakened. Want it with all your heart. The more you truly want to awaken, the more you will truly awaken. Instead of little awakenings, you can have big ones, saving yourself much time.

Today, keep awakening as your foremost goal. Want it with all your heart. Want to awaken from this dream of pain with every fiber of your being.

Lesson 36 – The Implications of Projection

At university, I studied a great deal of philosophy, which at its deepest level presents models of how reality works. By the end of my bachelor's degree, I was swimming in world views. I, myself, favored the existential perspective, which was heroic and artistic. But not quite half way into my senior year, I had a precocious thought, which was to examine all the world views from the perspective of which held the highest reward. With all the possibilities, it seemed clear that the choice for me came down to either the existential or the cosmic. As I considered these world views, the choice went 'hands down' to looking at the world from a spiritual perspective. Suddenly, I moved from the heroic-artistic but meaninglessness world of existentialism, to the renewed meaning that came from embracing a spiritual perspective.

As I moved past the hallowed halls of university and into the world, I became more and more interested in what created change and helped people out of suffering. This was why I appreciated *A Course in Miracles* when I discovered it. It not only contained the most thrilling work I had ever read in Psychology, Philosophy and Theology, it was practical. I not only experienced actual benefit for myself, but I was able to help many people as a result of it. The principles of *A Course in Miracles* worked on an everyday level. I was inspired by these principles to develop many techniques, one of the most powerful of which was projection.

In some earlier lessons from the 'Healing Pain Series', I have already discussed how, at the root of any problem, there is a grievance. The anger of the grievance is turned both outward and inward. The evidence of the grievance may be repressed so that we may not have an awareness of it within us.

I once worked with a woman in China who described her sister as quite toxic. We did a simple projection exercise of noticing what the perception was, pulling back the projection, recognizing whether she did the same things as her sister or compensated for these behaviors. For the most part, this woman had compensated for these behaviors and was at first indignant that I would suggest she had these self-concepts within her as shadow figures. Once she recognized the behaviors as her own self-concepts, then came the simple choice. I showed her how she was torturing herself for these behaviors, but she now had the choice to either keep torturing herself, or free herself from the torture chambers and go help her sister. With each projection, the woman chose to go help someone who was role playing her sister. Later, the woman reported to me that for two months afterwards her sister was a miraculously changed person. After the two months she developed other toxic behaviors, though never as bad as before.

I have seen numerous examples of a spouse finally stopping their physical, emotional or mental abuse when the client I was working with healed their own self-attack pattern. By eschewing guilt and taking personal responsibility instead, it gives us the possibility and the power to change ourselves, the other and the situation, because it is only a projection from our own mind.

We have hidden so much from ourselves under layers of dissociation and denial that we really believe that what we experience in the world is something real in its own right, rather than a projection on our part. Yet, in terms of the projection principle, what we see we believe, because we have projected it. This means whatever we see and experience, we already believe about ourselves. We have judged and rejected a part of ourselves, split it off from our conscious mind, repressed it and projected it out on someone or some thing.

This means that in the final essay, the person we have the grievance with, the one with whom we are really having trouble, is ourself. In their attack on us, others reflect our lack of self-love, our self-attack and even our self-hatred. These people are our own shadow figures. They are our own self-concepts – parts of our mind buried within. That is why all forgiveness is also self-forgiveness.

As *A Course in Miracles* states, "What you project, you believe." We believe what we project, and have already condemned and attacked it within us as we condemn and attack someone outside ourselves. And we feel righteous in doing so.

In truth, you are shadow boxing. You are only fighting the person in the mirror, and you know what's going to happen if you break that mirror. It is time to realize who you are really fighting. It is time to give up the self-attack and self-conflict that led to your trouble outside in the world and now with your body.

Today, bless yourself and everyone who seems to go against you. Realize that you must give up your self-attack to be healthy and at peace with the world inside and out.

Imagine those you hate or are angry with, standing in front of you. Write down the qualities you cannot stand in them. These are qualities you hate in yourself. You may notice that you have some of these same behaviors yourself or, on the other hand, you may have hidden them and acted in exactly the opposite way. If you have compensated in that way and then denied it to yourself, you will feel angry and insulted that anyone suggests you are like the person you hate.

Imagine these behaviors as yours. Accept them. Forgive them and yourself. Let go of these behaviors as being no big deal. Bless them and integrate back into you the energy that has supported negative self-concepts, so that it can be used positively. If you do this, then you will see the other person in a totally new way. You will have freed them and yourself.

Today, pick three people you are angry with or judging, and practice accepting them. Forgive them and yourself. Let go of these behaviors as being no big deal. Condemn neither them nor yourself. What you can consciously release in them, you will release in yourself in the unconscious. Bless them and integrate the energy. In this way, you declare the innocence of both.

Now pick three people from the past and do the same exercise.

Lesson 37 – Healing What is Not Whole

"When a brother perceives himself as sick, he is perceiving himself as NOT WHOLE, and therefore IN NEED."

A Course in Miracles

For someone to experience pain, they must first experience need. Without need, there is nothing to resist in life to cause the pain. Pain, therefore, represents a double fracture. The first comes from an incident of lost bonding, which puts us in a position where we experience ourselves as needy and are attempting to get something to make up for it. To attempt to **get** something is a form of resistance that can lead to us being defeated. Our attempting to **get** generates its own resistance in an area we could simply allow ourselves to receive, but our lost bonding has given us a split mind about receiving and a feeling of unworthiness. Otherwise, it would be easy to have anything that we wanted. With a split mind, we are afraid we won't get what we need, and we are afraid we will get it. The hurt or setback that comes from the defeat of trying to **get** is now compounded and increases our resistance.

At the deepest level of the mind, there is the primordial experience of separation or loss of Oneness. This led to soul patterns of lost bonding which in turn led to the resistance and dissociation. Separation leads to failure in our attempt to get our needs met. This occurs because of our inability to receive. This arises from the split mind, which comes from the conflict that led to lost bonding. Interrupt this pattern anywhere along the line, and you can stop the pain.

Heal the resistance, and you will stop the pain.

Heal the need, and you will heal what led to the pain.

Heal the separation, and you restore the bonding.

Heal the original separation, and you restore the awareness of Oneness that was lost at the beginning of time.

Let us now heal, layer by layer, the needs that come from separation, bringing greater wholeness with each.

This exercise is one that can go back to heal the deepest roots of separation, which led to pain. Let us first begin with healing the hurt that led to the pain.

If you were to know when that hurt first began, it was probably

If you were to know, who was a part of the situation when you suffered hurt and defeat, it was probably

What you were trying to get from them was probably

It is impossible to feel hurt unless you are trying to take something. What is it you are called to give this person instead? Ask this intuitively, as it may be a soul level gift that you have yet to bring out. Imagine yourself opening up this gift and sharing it with the one you were trying to get something from, and you will find the hurt or a layer of it disappearing.

For the next level, ask yourself when the original need began that led to the attempt to get something, and who was involved. Once again, ask yourself what need you were trying to get and, instead, what gift you brought in at a soul level to restore the bonding with this person. Share this gift energetically with them.

Now go back to that place where you experienced a great loss in your life. Imagine the light that is within you as spirit, and extend it to all of the people and things around you. Repeat this exercise until the scene becomes completely joyful or turns to light.

Repeat these exercises with any painful situation, past or present.

In a similar way, you can go back to the experience of the Fall where our dream of separation began. Sit quietly and ask for Heaven's help to awaken you by reconnecting you with the Love and Light that is Oneness. Any success in this area will restore you to joy, instead of the separation of your ego which breeds pain.

Lesson 38 – Free of Guilt, Free of Pain

We could never suffer pain without guilt of some kind. We punish ourselves for all the things we feel bad about. The extent that we feel bad about something is the extent we have not learned a certain lesson. As a result, when we attempt to push forward, we are plagued with heaviness and self-attack. We could change all of this by simply acknowledging that the guilt that is now generating pain in our lives is a mistake.

Pain is not God's Will for us. It is our ego's will, and our ego tells us that punishment is God's Will for us. We tell God not to worry about it and take care of the punishment ourselves. Guilt and self-punishment cannot be true spiritually because they are destructive, physically and psychologically. This could not be the Will of God, Who only wants what a loving Father would want for us. Guilt and self-punishment build our egos. God would not foster the illusion of the ego or guilt and pain, the illusions that build the ego. This is obviously the work of our ego. Let us commit to letting go of any guilt we discover. Anything that feels bad is guilt. This means that any negative emotion also carries the feelings of guilt.

The following is an excellent exercise for finding guilt in order to let go of it.

Recognize that any bad feeling from the past is now also guilt. Old hurts, heartbreaks, loss, shame, trauma that you carry inside make you feel bad, and when you feel bad about anything, it is guilt and you punish yourself for it. Begin first with your original family. Simply repeat this question to yourself over and over and see what pops up. Commit to let go of any guilt you discover.

In regard to my family, what I feel bad about is

After you have asked this question over a dozen times and nothing finally comes up, then ask yourself,

"Do I want to feel guilty or do I want all this to be healed now? Do I want to keep feeling bad and punish myself, or do I want to feel love instead?"

Choose to let go of all the bad feeling simply by putting it in God's Hands for dispersal.

Now choose another category, like relationships. After that, you can go through areas such as sex, money, competition, integrity, physical or emotional bullying, work, school, health, purpose, manipulation, etc. Remember, even when you were victimized you felt *bad*, but you also had to be feeling bad before you were victimized because victimization is a common form of self-punishment.

Then go through people: partner, Mom, Dad, siblings, children, relatives, schoolmates, friends, work associates, old romance or sex partners, abortions, deaths, etc.

Again after each category, choose to let go of the bad feeling simply by putting it all in God's Hands. This can save you the pain that occurs from self-punishment, as it is released in the easiest possible way.

Lesson 39 – No More Pain

Have you ever reached a place where you were so fed up by what was happening that something deep inside you snapped and you uttered a silent, "No more," with all the power of your heart and mind welded into your will. From that day and from that time, you never allowed yourself to fall back into whatever it was that you had resolutely stepped out of. I knew a nine-year-old First Nation's boy who marched into the room of the man who had been abusing and raping him almost every night of the week, and said the same thing with such finality that it stopped. Later that week he was beaten to within an inch of his life by a gang sent after him by the proctor and spent six months in the hospital, but he had finally had enough of the sexual abuse and said, "No more!"

Now it is time to invoke your power. Use the power of your mind. Use all the will your heart can summon and say, "No more! This is not God's Will for me and neither is it my own. I will be free of this."

Weld your heart and mind into one force and use it on your own behalf: One heart, one mind, one will, united with God's Will:

"No More!"

Let this be your anthem. Let this be your mantra. Let these be your words of power.

"No more! I will be free!"

Lesson 40 – See Yourself as God Sees You

To see ourself as God sees us is to know ourself as the precious child of God. God sees us as deserving every good thing. He could not wish pain on us and remain a loving father, and He is a Loving Father. When we left the paradise of Oneness, our separation made the dark emotions of guilt. Not being able to stand the guilt or the separation, we projected that it was God who threw us out of the Garden and was cruel to us. But the force of Love that is God could never do such a thing and remain either the force of Love or God. Our guilt made a world of punishment, and in that world we have crucified ourselves. Yet, in our belief that God threw us out of paradise into a world of pain and death, we have cut ourselves off from Him. But God as Perfection could only create what was perfect and so could not, and did not, make a world of death. He wants only our remembrance and return to Oneness as we feel the irresistible pull of love to Love that will eventually unite us.

Today, see yourself as God sees you, innocent and loved. Let it be so. Feel God's love. Feel what you deserve. Know yourself as God's precious child nestled in his Being.

Lesson 41 – The Crossroads of Life and Death

Over the years, I have worked with a number of people with catastrophic illness or who have a strong death temptation. Years ago I came up with an exercise to measure a person's attitude toward life or death. A person's attitude is crucial in that it is the direction they are heading. If they are heading toward death without fully realizing this, then it is time for them to recognize what they are doing and make a new choice. You can do this on your own, mustering as much will as possible for a new and truer choice, or you can do this by asking for Heaven's help.

Imagine the grid on this page

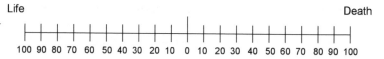

Now, as you look at the grid, imagine you can see where you are and whether you are heading toward life or death. Which do you want it to be? Choose that. Commit to that. Want that with your whole heart. Integrate any hidden or not so hidden parts that are self-destructive with the parts that are positive and want to make a new beginning. Ask for and receive Heaven's help in your choice for life.

Lesson 42 – Pain as a Defense

Both physical and emotional pain are defenses the ego uses to protect itself. Pain serves to defend the ego by attacking us. It defends against the direction that would free us and against the gift that hides under the conflict that is generating the pain. In a conflict, two parts of our mind are pushing against each other in the most unpleasant of ways.

Pain is a distraction, and it is the most consuming type of distraction. Almost always, our attention goes to our pain and, in this way, the ego has succeeded in delaying us. Yet, if we were to take a moment to realize how our pain is being used by the ego against us, we would begin to realize that the ego is not our friend, and we no longer need honor the contract we have made with it. If we further examined this contract, we would realize that it ends in our demise, orchestrated by the ego.

After years of instilling in us the vicious circle of superiority-inferiority, the ego finally begins to believe it is too good even for us. If we read the small print on our contract with the ego, we would realize that it is entirely bogus, and the ego gave us nothing that really made us happy. It was meant to help us navigate in this world, but it was also meant to let go of its control at about the age of eighteen or nineteen. It simply never let go.

If you are in pain, ask for the way out and allow your intuition to show you the path to freedom. Ask for the gift the ego has hidden, embrace that and let it bring the peace that has been waiting for you. Pain reduces us to the physical and the emotional aspects of our life, but the spiritual trumps this. Ask what Heaven has for you that would bless you and bring surcease of pain. Both truth and Heaven are on your side.

Lesson 43 – Pain Results When the Flow is Stopped

When the flow is stopped, it is because too much conflict or resistance has built up. There are some things that can serve to put us back in the flow in such a way as to relieve the pain. The most effective thing I found in this regard is giving. By listening a moment within, we can discover who needs our help and who we are called to give to, and what we are called to give to them. Sometimes the amount of blockage is so severe that this may need to be repeated, but it is an easy exercise. While my field of study is not as extensive with people in physical pain, I have seen this particular exercise work on people in the most dire emotional pain there is. People who have used it for physical pain have reported varying degrees of success.

Another way to re-establish the flow is to express gratitude and appreciation toward those around us, especially to those who 'pop' into our minds intuitively when we ask who to express gratitude or appreciation toward.

Forgiveness is another major way to re-establish the flow. As the flow is blocked by guilt, judgment, grievance and self-attack, forgiveness is the perfect antidote to such mistakes. Forgiveness frees us and the one we forgive. Ask who it is you are called to forgive and ask for Heaven's grace to help accomplish it. If you are attacking yourself, forgiveness of others releases you also. Forgive the pain and anyone or anything that comes to your mind.

Trust is another way to free us of the blockages that are stopping the flow, as trust, like forgiveness, heals the fear under every place the flow is stopped.

Love and willingness also heal fear, so if we give our love to those around us and send our love to those who pop into our mind, it can move us back into the flow. Willingness also moves us forward where fear had stopped us. The greater the pain, the greater the fear. Willingness will move us forwards, and when there is great pain, great willingness helps us leap forward to the next chapter in our life. Receiving can also unblock the flow. Receive what Heaven wants to give you. Pain and blockage is not Heaven's Will for you. It will supply an antidote if you are open to it.

Gifts are another way to re-establish the flow. What gifts does Heaven want to give you to replace your pain? Receive these. What gift are you called to give to another? Intuit who the person is, and what the gift is that you are called to give them. Imagine yourself opening up this gift in your mind. Then embrace and share it with them with love.

Lesson 44 – The Search for Roots

I have found that our traumatic, painful events have been planned by us at a soul level. This is our unconscious or soul-mind. Our traumas are the result of unfinished business that we have carried, lessons that we set up to learn in this life. What is still unfinished, and is either buried or so big that it could not have been dealt with in any other way, comes to us in the form of a traumatic event. This releases the emotion and unfinished lesson buried deep within our mind. When such emotions come to the surface, they bring with them both guilt and the indirect guilt that comes from all the negative emotions. These make us feel bad and have the same dark effect as guilt. So what may have begun as a heartbreak or loss then gets attached to guilt, generating vicious downward circles of self-punishment. We all have these pockets of buried pain, resistance and guilt repressed within us. If we didn't, we would already have attained not just happiness but enlightenment and Oneness.

We know when unconscious pain surfaces, which is what psychiatry refers to as primary process, because we hurt so badly it takes us to our knees. Let me enumerate some of the pockets of unconscious pain that I have discovered. After visiting these places numerous times with clients, I began to recognize them by the names that they have been given: the Ocean of Sadness, the Great Fears, Shamanic Tests, the Abyss, Sacred Fire Pain, the Great Wars, Valuelessness, Failure, Mastery Level Tests, the Graveyard, the Void, the Hells, Dark Nights of the Soul, Meaninglessness, Dark Stories, 'Other Lifetimes', Conspiracies, Shadows, Ancestral Patterns, Core Authority Conflict Issues, Tantrums, 'Shticks,' Idols, the Collective Unconscious, the Collective Ego, the Astral, and the primordial pain that came from the first separation or 'the Fall.'

Our ego thrives on all that generates pain. Pain distracts us from life, our purpose and the grace being given to us. When we are taken to our knees with pain, our ability to concentrate dissolves. Now with all of these painful karmic traps, which are the patterns of actions from the past, it is easy to get confused. Even Krishna was said to have remarked that he got confused about the sixty-four karmas. Many thousands of years ago the Hindus discovered these karmas are the roots and patterns of what creates problems for us.

Most people do not need to know exactly where each issue is coming from. They just want to stop the pain. For them, I would suggest a simple letting go. It is this:

I place my pain in the Hands of God.

I place my fear in the Hands of God.

I place my mistaken choices from both past and present in the Hands of God.

I place whatever roots there are to this pain in the Hands of God.

I place my mind in the Hands of God.

I place my future in the Hands of God.

You could also simply choose to **let go** of:

1. Your pain
2. Your mistaken choices
3. The roots of this pain

Then choose the truth for yourself and your future.

For those who like to find the roots of their issues, choose a number between one and twenty-three. Now choose a second number between one and twenty-three. Finally choose a third number between one and twenty-three.

Here are what the numbers reflect:

1. *The Ocean of Sadness* – A huge pocket of unconscious loss and sadness covered over by our self-concepts.
2. *The Great Fears* – These are the fears, terrors and other emotions associated with our greatest fears which are relegated to the unconscious.
3. *Shamanic Test* – We venture everything to reach a new stage of consciousness if we succeed. If we fail, it feels like our heart is being ripped out.
4. *The Abyss* – One of the deep, dark and frightening places of emptiness within, that seems to have no end.
5. *Sacred Fire Pain* – The pain is so great we are on our knees. It comes from core splits in the mind.

6. *Valuelessness and Primordial Failure* – Great pockets of primordial guilt.

7. *The Graveyard* – This is where we have buried selves and even parts of selves that have died.

8. *The Void* – This is an even deeper black hole in the mind than the abyss.

9. *The Hells* – These are places of profound torment and self-torture, deep within the mind.

10. *Dark Stories* – These are the dark and painful scripts that **we** have been writing.

11. *'Other Lifetimes'* – These are the soul patterns affecting us now that we haven't healed yet. Whether they are metaphoric stories that the mind made up, as we do in a dream, or an actual fact is for you to decide.

12. *Conspiracies* – These are traps set up by us for some mistaken payoff, and now it looks like there is no way out.

13. *Shadows* – Aspects or mistaken beliefs about ourselves that we repress but still punish ourselves for. We judge something in us, split it off, repress it and project it on others.

14. *Ancestral Patterns* – Unresolved pain and conflict passed down through our family from our ancestors.

15. *Idols* – Things we have made into false gods. We think they will save us and make us happy.

16. *Tantrums* – Using dark emotions or negative experience to complain profoundly in an immature fashion.

17. *'Shticks'* – A game you are playing at an unconscious level that punishes yourself and others. It is typically full of passive-aggression.

18. *Rebelliousness* – Core authority conflict.

19. *Meaninglessness* – Without love and Heaven's meaning, there is only the meaning that we have assigned to the world to cover its meaninglessness.

20. *Dark Night of the Soul* – Places of deep suffering and utter darkness where we no longer experience God. The first one began with the Fall.

21. *Primordial Pain* – This is pain that comes from our first imagined splits from Oneness. The 'Fall' from Oneness led to the physical universe and a belief in the body as our identity. It is a level of agony and anguish.

22. *The Collective Ego* – The principle of separation, specialness and competition. These principles bring all the pain as it exists in the universe.

23. *The Astral* – Aspects of the ancient ego that fight to dominate, possess and delay the joining-healing process that leads to Oneness. It contains the dark energy of the demonic and dark gods.

Now let go of whichever of the dynamics you picked. Put them in the Hands of God or give them to your higher mind to heal.

Lesson 45 – Claiming a Painfree Life

Many times pain makes us lose our focus, rendering us weak and vulnerable. This is part of the ego's use of pain. All of our attention goes to the pain, leaving us dull and haphazard in regard to our life. We've taken a hit, but we're trying to go forward. Pain disconnects us from ourselves, as well as disconnecting us from grace and its power. But if we are aware of this, we can act in such a way as to counter it. In so doing we can muster up the courage to focus our power to claim that our mind be free.

Claiming is a power of the mind that commands that what belongs to us be ours. It calls for what we deserve. We can claim all of our focus and power back and not be at the effect of pain. We can claim grace and Heaven's help. We can claim anything we find at all believable. For instance, if we believe that the pain can end immediately, claim that. If not, claim the faith to accomplish it. We can claim what our mind can accept. We can claim that the pain lessens every day or that they find a drug or treatment that assuages our pain and ends our malady.

My wife had a chronic neck problem since a ski accident thirty years ago, but lately she seemed to reach a level of consciousness that allowed us to find a chiropractor who did such excellent work that she became pain free. You can claim the level of consciousness needed so that you also can find who or what you need to liberate you from your yoke of pain. You deserve it. Claim what God wants to give you.

Claiming is one of the natural gifts of your mind. It is a power available to you, but only if you use it. Practice claiming until it becomes natural to you.

Lesson 46 – Radical Acceptance

Of course, you do not want to suffer. Yet, you do. You would like to be free of the pain but you are not. Now is the time to accept your condition – one of pain. Radical acceptance is a highly advanced spiritual technique to deal with pain. Do not seek to change it. Change is impossible. *You* cannot get yourself out of pain because the *you* that you believe you are, is not only in pain, it is pain. In such a condition only one thing is possible and that is acceptance. It is radical acceptance because you are probably in a situation that you would rather not be in. Now it is time to stop resisting. It has not succeeded. There is one possibility left for success and that is to accept your situation and accept your pain. It is not your first choice now. It is your only choice. Stop fighting against what is occurring. Accept it. Accept it radically. This is the way it is. This is how it will always be. Don't fight it. Don't give up either. Accept it. All kinds of emotions may surface. Accept them. Feel them. Fly through them by experiencing them totally. Embrace them. Go no further. Be willing to have this be the way it is, forever.

The paradox of acceptance is that only when there is total acceptance can something new happen. So totally accept your pain. Stop trying to avoid it. Go into it. This is the way it is so you might as well ride the horse in the direction it is going. Be brave about it. Feel it. Feel every nuance of it. Accept it as it is. Your acceptance allows you to handle it. So handle it. What you accept, you are not stuck with. Have courage. Ask for Heaven's help. You break the ego's painful hold on you when you accept the situation as it is. You have been suffering so now instead of fighting it, simply be one with it. When you join with your experience, it unfolds but only when you enter it fully. Now is that time. This is the place. There is nowhere to run and nowhere to hide. Be one with what is. Experience your own experience. Feel what you are feeling in a wholehearted way. It is the only way out. You must enter into it fully. When you do, you will once again move out of this place where you are stuck.

What are you waiting for? Now is the time of release. Radically accept what is happening emotionally and physically. You might as well; it is the only thing happening. Acceptance is the only way out. It is the alternative to the hidden conflict that keeps you suffering and will never release you. Accept your pain now. Do it with Heaven's help. Move into it and you can move through it. Acceptance brings flow. Conflict both generates pain and stops you from going forward. Radical acceptance unravels the conflict into flow.

Lesson 47 – *What Misery Hides*

When we suffer, our awareness shrinks and it is all we can do to handle the misery. Our mind contracts; our world contracts. Our mind is taken up by the pain. While great pain can occur at any stage of growth, as we reach into higher levels of consciousness the ego uses misery to block our forward progress. If you are in devastating misery, you may want to explore what it hides. Because if you know what it hides, it can be healed. Knowing the problem is half the battle. We have already explored how pain and problems hide gifts. The greater the pain, the greater the gift it hides.

As I was exploring the Unity level of consciousness, I began to see that it was defended by extreme levels of suffering. Unity is the level of consciousness in which we begin to experience more and more of the interconnectedness of all things. As I began to explore the devastation, utter loneliness, alienation and misery blocking the Unity level, I discovered that, at a deeper level, it was hiding and expressing a tantrum. Misery complains in a vocal and painful way about our suffering. Metaphorically, we throw ourselves down on the floor, suffering greatly because some need we have is not being met. And we are willing to suffer to make the point. Let us take a moment and reflect about our misery being a tantrum.

All problems are a form of complaint, but extreme suffering reflects a tantrum. What is your tantrum about and who is it directed towards? What need was not met for you? Whose attention are you trying to get? Who is it you are complaining to that they have done you wrong? Whoever it is, you are bitter about some need not being met. You are refusing to get over it and grow up, in the hope that your tantrum might be the way to get your need met. While this is unconscious, it is no less devastating to your life.

Once you have awareness about this tantrum there will be flow and even excitement, if you do not attack yourself about it, which is an ego ploy to keep it. Yet this is not the end of what is making the misery, there is a deeper level. If you fully delve into your tantrum, you will begin to realize that it is hiding a 'shtick'. This Yiddish word describes a level of tantrum that is destructive and self-destructive. It is typically both immature and passive-aggressive. It is quite defensive, attacking outwardly and when confronted attacking inwardly. Symptoms may be pain, illness, insanity, failure, etc. It hides the glee of the ego which is using the situation to win, building itself and defeating the people around you by making help impossible. This reflects the core authority conflict with God and hides the next layer of the mind which is rebellion. Who are you rebelling against? If you did not include God on your list, as well as a significant person around you, your list is incomplete. So dwell awhile on your pain being a form of rebellion. What are you rebelling about? Why did you choose to have it take this form? Do you want to continue this stance or make another choice?

You may want to examine what rebellion hides because, if you embrace what it hides, it quickly begins to dissolve the rebellion with its symptom of pain.

What rebellion hides is Unity – the interconnectedness of all things. This is a higher state of consciousness that helps dissolve your personal ego and displaces it from the throne it has put itself on through your mistaken choices. In Unity what you experience is the joy that comes from the relatedness of all things.

If you follow each step in your mind from misery, there is a groove that it follows. Misery unfolds to tantrum. Tantrums will lead you to the hidden 'shtick,' which leads you to rebellion. But if you don't stop there, what hides beneath this is the unity of all life and the joy that goes with it.

So follow this groove until you reach joy. You have nothing to lose but your pain.

Lesson 48 – Using Process Cards

How you perceive is how you experience. All healing then is a change of perception. As you change your mind, which is the cause, so do you change the world and your experience, which is the effect.

Since 1975, I have been studying process, which is how things unfold. I was supervised by two psychiatrists at the Naval Drug Rehabilitation Center and the first concept they introduced me to was that of psychological process. This is how things unfold in groups and individual sessions. Soon I discovered that process was similarly unfolding in life as well as in therapy. I also studied the I-Ching and Tarot, watching how these symbols synchronistically played a part, as they reflected how life unfolded. It was this that eventually led me to start developing Healing Cards that can be used to depict process as it unfolds in our lives and problems. I found that I could use symbols, in this case cards, to show the essence of what is occurring at our level.

As I worked with the process cards, I *discovered* that there might be one or more negative cards covering a positive card. This demonstrated positive process was the truth and that it was being covered over by some negative process. Negative process really didn't keep things from unfolding, it simply slowed and distracted from the positive process, while showing the painful regression that was occurring. This negative, painful regression was actually a defense against the truth. This was evidenced by the positive process card that the unfolding of negative process always led to.

I found that although these negative cards sometimes reflected deep subconscious or unconscious traps, they could be easily dismissed, or let go of, as they were simply defenses. They weren't the truth. They weren't what was really going on. They concealed the positive process. When they were let go of the next layer emerged, either positive or negative. We could keep letting go of negative process until we reached the positive process, as reflected by the card. Then we could embrace the positive process, jump into it as if it was a river, or let it pour through us to move life forward naturally and easily.

Once you have reached the level of positive process, you could pull another card to show what gift you have for yourself today to help with a problem. If you get a negative card in this pick, it means you brought in a healing gift in this regard. So if you pulled the *Guilt* card, for instance, it means your gift for yourself today is *Healing Guilt*. Whatever card you then pull for your gift to yourself, whether positive or negative, is positive when showing you your gift. You can imagine if you like going to that place in your mind where your gifts wait in potential. There are thousands of gifts there, but one door will be glowing. Open that door and embrace the gift. Let it flow through you and into your life.

The next card to pull is the gift that Heaven has for you to help in this situation and, of course, it is always positive. If it's a negative card, it means you are given the healing of that particular negativity. Either way, positive or the healing of the negative, receive this card for yourself and your life.

You can use healing cards to ask specific questions and, as you learn to relate to the cards, they have a stronger and stronger impact. Some people, of course, take to the cards quickly and easily as if they have been doing them all their lives. As process is the heart of what is going on in a situation, it's helpful to have cards, especially to show what is happening at subconscious and unconscious levels.

But cards are not necessary. You can simply reflect on the flow of what is occurring. The major traps that stop the flow are dependency, power struggle and pairing. Dependency is when we lean on another to get our needs met. In this case, life will not unfold unless, of course, the giver is giving love as well as caretaking. The fight and flight of power struggle also reflects an experience of fear where life is not unfolding. Pairing, which is the specialness that excludes others, can also stop the unfolding in a group. Love, on the other hand, would make the couple more available to everyone in love. You can reflect on what is occurring. If it is positive, embrace it. If it is negative, realize it is not the truth and let it go.

You could ask Universal Inspiration what is going on in your situation that has led to your current problem and reflect on the process, or pull process cards - letting go of the negative until you reach the positive. If you have three or more negative cards or layers of negativity before you reach the positive card, it means you have set up a conspiracy which is a trap so big it looks as if there is no way out. If there are seven or more negative process cards, it is a place of shattered dreams which we usually defend by adamantly refusing to change, out of some fear, or because we would have to deal with the negative emotion. Of course, pulling these process cards, or reflecting on your process, shows that you are now ready to address this area. Simply let go of each negative layer, as reflected by the cards or the process, until you no longer feel any attachment or resistance to the negative process. If you put the negative process in God's Hands, you know that it will be taken care of for you. Let go of all the negative process until you come to what is really going on. Then, feel the flow of that positive process through yourself.

When you are ready, pull the card or reflect on what your soul brought in as a gift for just this situation. Embrace and enjoy this. Next, pull a card for Heaven's gift to you and receive that. This just shows what is available to you in the way of grace.

You can pull healing cards about what is unfolding for your friends. Since all minds are connected, and at an unconscious level they are just reflecting your mind, you can pull process cards for them, letting go of what is not positive. In the same way, you can pull cards regarding the gift you brought in to help them and even receive Heaven's gift for them. They may be able to resist Heaven, but not you. Receive the gift for them and then share your and Heaven's gift energetically with them.

There are many questions you could ask for yourself or a friend, such as what would it take for you to achieve a miracle in this situation. Then pull your process and gift cards or simply use your intuition as your higher mind has all of these answers.

You can use any Tarot or card pack if you know the meaning of the symbols. Or you can order the Psychology of Vision Process Cards at **www.pov-int.com**. There are card packs in English, German and one in Mandarin.

The following decks are available:

Enlightenment Pack, a general set of healing cards.

Romance and Relationship Deck, as part of the Relationship Series.

Life Stories Deck

Conspiracy Deck

Archetypes and Shadows Deck, part of the Unconscious Series.

In German, there are six card decks including the Life Story Cards which reflect the key soul stories we tell over and over again.

These decks can be all used together, or in part if you like. The beauty of the cards is that they can pull up what's stopping you below the level of the conscious mind.

If you do not have cards and would like to begin right away, then you can use your intuition or get a tarot deck or a regular deck of cards with a book to explain the symbols. Use these to feel and recognize what is going on at each level until you get to your positive process. Accept your healing gift for yourself, as well as Heaven's gift for you. This can all serve to get you back in the flow.

For very chronic issues or pain, I would suggest that you follow this healing regimen with the process cards for twenty-two days straight. The cards are simple and straightforward, which is of great use in healing what we have hidden from ourselves. You can consciously let go of what you do not want.

Again, as an alternative, you can work without the cards simply tuning in to what the process is. You can become quite astute as you study this process and of course, some of you have a natural awareness of what is unfolding if you turn your mind in this direction.

Lesson 49 – *Attacking Yourself*

The greatest human addiction is attacking ourselves. We attack ourselves when we feel bad. We attack ourselves when we feel good. We punish ourselves when we feel guilt and we punish ourselves when we lose. With every negative emotion that we feel, there is also self-attack. Any problem, accident, setback or pain is a form of self-attack. Every self-concept or personality we have within us pushes and protects its directives with self-attack. We have many thousands of self-concepts, many of which are so contradictory that there is no way we can get it right. We have to dissociate most of the self-attack we have or, as *A Course in Miracles* states, we'd go running off a cliff. In spite of numbing the wound, we are still bleeding from it.

Think of the children you love the most. Would you want them to attack themselves like that? If you wouldn't want the people you love the most attacking themselves like that, then you'd better give up your addiction to attacking yourself.

After studying the phenomenon of self-attack for six months, I found that the purpose the ego had for this self-attack was to build and strengthen itself rather than step forward to greater success and less ego. It also used self-attack to get us distracted and self-obsessed to the point that we could not hear the calls for help coming from those we love or those who needed us. Our self-attack is made to keep us separate and out of the flow. If we gave up our self-attack, or even stepped through it to reach out to another in support, both of us would go into flow. Helping others, helps us. Attacking ourself attacks everyone we love because as *A Course in Miracles* states, "Attack is not discrete." We can't get away with only attacking ourselves; we attack everyone we love and who loves us, if only by our withdrawal from them in attacking ourselves.

Self-attack can be subtle. It hides under self-consciousness and embarrassment. It hides under our grievances and judgments. It hides under fears, worries, upsets and concerns. Fear comes from attack thoughts within us. Whatever we do to another we do to ourselves first. When we send out judgment and attack thoughts, we see the same coming back to us. So when we have fear, it shows that we are attacking ourselves.

You deserve every tender mercy. Your ego, which builds itself through your self-attack, is not your friend.

Categorically give up your self-attack and be compassionate to yourself. When you catch yourself wanting to attack yourself ask, "Who needs my help?" Whoever pops into your mind is the person to send love to. This will help both of you.

Give up your grievances. They are killing you. Give up your judgments. They are the root of all your suffering. Give up your fear, it attacks you as well as the world around you.

Here's an exercise from *A Course in Miracles* that will help you become aware of your attack thoughts. Think of situations that are a problem or a concern to you.

Ask yourself, "In the situation regarding _____, I'm afraid _____ will happen. This thought is a thought I'm using to attack myself. I choose not to do that any more.

Instead, I will send love to _____ who needs my help".

Do the exercises with each of these problems or areas of concern until no more worries come forth. Then move on to the next. It's better to do ten, one or two minute exercises throughout the day, than to try to do it all at once. This is an excellent lesson to continue for the next week to help free yourself of your self-attack.

Help your brothers and sisters by supporting them when they want to attack themselves. When you have dropped the knife in your hands which you have used to carve canyons out of your heart, then with authority, you can reach for the knife in theirs.

Lesson 50 – Seeing Clearly

Any problem, such as pain, reflects a level of untruth. Pain is not Heaven's Will for us, nor is it our true will. This means that underneath our suffering there is a true process. This is loving and happy compared with the painful process we have gotten caught up in. We can change our perception and recognize the true and pain-free process that is unfolding right now in our lives.

There is an exercise I learned from *A Course in Miracles* that is one of my favorites as I have found it effective in changing my perspective of a perceived problem.

You simply imagine your painful situation. Muster all your will and, as you gaze at the scene, state to yourself with all your heart, "I am determined to see." Then simply notice any shifts in your experience, visually or emotionally. Once again, repeat the words, "I am determined to see." And simply notice any shifts in feeling or perception. Keep repeating this simple but transformative exercise, over and over again until you have reached peace.

You may want to get comfortable and play some music as you do this. Recognize that your pain did not just come out of nowhere. It is the fruit of a tree that has deep roots.

Choose three major incidents that you feel had a direct or ancillary influence on the stress and pain in your life now. Repeat this exercise, saying," I am determined to see this differently", until you reach a place of peace and ease with each of these incidents.

Finally, choose three major incidents from the past, and with all the will your heart can call upon, state toward each one "I want to see this situation with _____ differently".

After each statement, witness the changes that occur. Allow this unfolding to occur until the situation has become happy.

"I am determined to see this situation with _____ differently." Then measure each situation with the truth and watch your perception unfold until there is only peace.

Lesson 51 – The Layers of Pain

Pain is often layered, so that as we work through one layer of resistance in our healing, we are still not free of the pain. Pain shows resistance to some person or situation. Resistance in regard to a situation can be made up of many relationships, from either the past or present.

Given these principles there are two ways to approach your pain. One is to use your intuition and ask yourself how many layers of resistance need to be healed for you to be pain free. The other is simply to begin healing each layer of pain until you are free.

To begin the healing process start with the first layer and ask who this layer has to do with. Whoever comes to mind, set out to join with this person, mind to mind. Move through the grievances and the emotional distance until you reach a place of peace with them. Joining is simply moving with love toward another until all the emotion, judgment and pain has dissolved and finally your two minds have become one. Ask your own higher mind to help in this process, as its function is to help you heal. When you have finally become one mind with this person, ask yourself who there is at the next layer to heal with, and repeat the joining process. It does not matter whether you take a long time or a short time. You will find your own stride and be heading in a healing direction. You may also find that a person comes up in more than one layer. You may be working through different layers of emotions, judgments and resistances. Simply trust your process until you become one with this person.

This person represents your self-concepts. As you join with them, your self-concepts are integrated into a new wholeness. Later other issues or self-concepts may also be projected onto the same person. So, as you go deeper, you will find new or old judgments on them. Your resistance on the outside to this person, shows you the pain you have on the inside. This typically stems from conflicts that were in place even before you met this person. Now you can use the outside situation to heal both the inner and the outer levels, which are actually the same.

You can use the power of joining to heal your mind and heal your pain as it makes your relationships and your mind whole. Today, and for the next week, practice healing your layers of resistance and your relationships through joining.

Lesson 52 – The Purpose of Pain

We are creatures of purpose. Everything serves a purpose for us, even if we don't think there is any purpose to our suffering. If we don't understand how everything serves a purpose for us, we don't really understand psychology. Once I understood that this was how our mind worked, I reached a whole new level of effectiveness in my healing work.

It is important to ask yourself what purpose this pain serves for you:

- What is your payoff?
- What need are you trying to get met?
- What does it allow you to do?
- How does this pain feed your need for significance?
- What is it that you don't have to do as a result of the pain?
- What fear are you trying to protect?
- Who is your fear of intimacy with?
- What attachment is this pain an attempt to hold onto?
- What are you afraid would happen at the next step?
- What is your fear of success about?
- What is it you are afraid to lose?
- What do you get to be right about by having this pain?
- What is it that your ego has offered you if only you'd suffer a little pain to get it?
- What is your pain trying to prove?
- Who is your authority conflict with?
- Who are you trying to defeat, that you are willing to suffer in order to win?

These are but a few of the questions you could ask yourself. If you don't like the answers you pull out of your subconscious, you could change your mind. You could see a world different to the one you see. You could choose again. It is best to answer these questions intuitively or to dwell on each one until your answer emerges. There is an answer to every question. If you don't like your answers, you could give them to your higher mind to transform and have the truth put in its place.

Lesson 53 – Joining

Joining is both a method and a way of life. Joining allows you not only to approach something but to enter it with your mind. In the case of another human being, you join them mind to mind. This can create what *A Course in Miracles* calls a "Holy Instant," which is a joining so profound it can lead to awakening, even at times to the experience of Oneness.

We have made a world of separation from our judgments and as *A Course in Miracles* states, "from judgment comes all the suffering of the world." Joining can become a way of life where you join with people, animals and even objects or situations. When you succeed, you have not only removed the distance presently between you, but also between aspects of your own mind. You gain a profound understanding and empathy with whoever or whatever you are joining with.

Your success in joining depends on your intention to succeed in becoming one with another. The space between you and the other is your judgment, your separation and your resistance. As you join, you are extending yourself in love and establishing bonding with the other. It is this **distance** that **holds your pain**. That is why it is so helpful to join with those you are most aggrieved with first, as this situation contains a great amount of emotional distance. Any joining that you do with another helps you move closer in love to yourself and everyone. Even if you do not attain a mystical state in joining, any success at all helps you open your heart, which is good on so many levels.

As you join with another, and move through layer after layer of resistance, you "burn" through layers of the pain inside you and create more openness. Sometimes as you join, you have a breakthrough and then you can feel the issue between you and another also moving up, chakra by chakra, breakthrough by breakthrough, to the fourteenth chakra, the seventh chakra above the head - achieving a miracle through your joining.

Do this exercise of joining for nine days, beginning on the first day with the person you love the most. Spend the day joining with them. Begin with loving them the first few minutes and then feel and sense yourself becoming one with this person. Spend fifteen minutes in the morning and evening sitting quietly joining them, mind to mind, as if you were one person in two bodies. During the day, join this person every time you think of them.

On the second day do this with the person you are having the biggest problem with.

On the third day, choose an animal.

On the fourth day, choose a political figure or world leader you admire.

On the fifth day, choose a political or world leader you have judgment on.

On the sixth day, choose an inanimate object.

On the seventh day, choose once more the person you are having the biggest problem with.

On the eighth day choose the person you love the most. It's fine to choose someone who has left their body.

On the ninth day, join with God.

Join for fifteen minutes in the morning and evening. Any extra time you can find to contribute to this exercise, either to lengthen the morning or evening sessions or have another session during the day, is most helpful, not only with lessening your pain, but with opening your heart, increasing your ability to receive, etc. Also, every time you think of the person, animal or thing, go to join them mind to mind. The more you join with another the more grace comes in.

This is a powerful exercise which is relatively simple. It can help you burn away resistance at the very least, and at best will open the possibility of an awakening experience. Wouldn't you want to commit to becoming an expert in this exercise? The more you practice it, the more you can open your heart and create bonding with a wide variety of people. This allows more ease, flow and understanding in your life.

Ask your higher mind for help each day, set your intention for the highest goals and commit to this exercise along with the healing and transcendence that come from joining. Your joining can be healing, mystical or miraculous and it opens your heart making you available for partnership.

Lesson 54 – Meditation on God

There is a meditation I learned from *The Disappearance of the Universe* by Gary Renard. It is a book I highly recommend. And I have found this meditation to be of good avail in times of difficulty. It also has the ability after a few days use to provide answers or direction as we need them.

It states in *A Course in Miracles* that we only have one real need and that is the need for God. In this 5-10 minute meditation, you imagine yourself in the Mind of God. Let all your cares, worries and pain seep out of you. Pain comes from separation. God is Love and Oneness. Do this meditation once in the morning and once at night and any time in between that you feel the need. This is worth getting up a few minutes early for in the morning if you have a busy schedule. You could see a Heavenly figure leading you into that center of the Mind of God. Let yourself be at peace. Float in that Love. Let yourself be restored.

This could be the most important time of your day. Give yourself the opportunity and let God do the rest.

Lesson 55 – The Conflict of Pain

When we are in pain, we do not want to be feeling pain. This puts us in conflict about the pain we are experiencing. We are at odds with our experience.

Yet, there is another layer of conflict that we are in. For us to experience pain, at least two parts of our mind must be in conflict. It is this conflict that generates not only a fear of moving forward, but also pain in the situation we are experiencing. Two parts of our mind are in power struggle, and neither will be satisfied until there is an integration of both parts.

Simple acceptance of the pain will not be enough to release us from pain if two of the *deeper parts of mind are still in conflict.*

If nothing else, you could ask your higher mind to identify and integrate the two parts of the mind in conflict. Ask your higher mind to accomplish this resolution for however many layers the conflict goes down. Often the conflict goes down, layer after layer, to a root conflict.

You can also do at least the first major layer of this integration yourself, by noticing that the more prominent part of your mind, the part you identify with, is in conflict with another more hidden part, usually represented by the outward form of the problem. You can begin to identify the more hidden aspect of the conflict by identifying the opposite to what is in your conscious mind.

There is some hidden attachment or need and we refuse to go forward without it being met. What is that attachment? What does the pain or problem show you?

To examine your subconscious, pretend you want the pain or problem. Why could you possibly want it? What could you possibly be trying to get from the pain or problem? What is it you could possibly be attached to? Imagine this hidden attachment, and the more prominent part you identify with, for however many levels the conflict goes down inside you. Melt both sides down to their pure energy and join them together in a whole.

While the pain has been helpful to point out the conflict, we do not like to suffer. So imagine the parts of you that are suffering, and the part that does not want to suffer, melting down to their pure energy and joining together. When there is wholeness, there is no pain, only a pleasant flow. Search for all your conflicts leading to your present pain and ask that they be integrated for you.

Invoke the Divine Presence so that the ability to find the hidden parts of the conflict, and having the parts integrated, becomes second nature to you with the help of grace. Move beyond your conflicts, into a new wholeness through Heaven's help.

Lesson 56 – Invulnerability

The more harmless we are in thought and behavior, the more invulnerable we become. The more benign we are in our thoughts, the happier we feel. If we have attack thoughts, we will have all kinds of emotions that are rife with pain and conflict. It is so easy to dissociate and be in denial but it is safe to say that any kind of negativity in thought, emotion or what happens to us comes from our attack thoughts. There is no separation, fear, guilt or authority conflict without attack thoughts on our part. Our attack thoughts lead to our own and others' negative experiences. We carry attack at subconscious, unconscious and primordial levels, reaping negative experience, but because it is buried under our denial, we are not aware of its source in our own mind. And while the root of our present pain may be ancestral, soul, the collective unconscious, the collective ego, the dark unconscious or the primordial separation, we can typically trace the present pain to a more recent root in our past. There will be an incident in this life in which the ancient pattern can show itself and be resolved.

When pain comes up, we can use it like a fireman uses a fire pole to get to the fire engine quickly. We can use the pain to trace back to the root of the pain.

Using your intuition, ask yourself:

If I were to know when the root of the emotional pain began that led to this current emotional or physical pain, it was probably at the age of

And it probably occurred with me and

In some cases, using this method can bring up things that did not happen as such, but it was some thought, fantasy or dream that programmed us as if it actually did happen.

When you get back to the "original incident," ask yourself what positive lesson you were looking to learn to get beyond the pain.

Ask yourself what gift you had within, at a soul level, that would have been the antidote to the situation back then, and helpful now. Also, ask what gift Heaven would have given you as the antidote to obviate that past situation gracefully.

Next, ask who, beside yourself, you were attacking to have that experience occur? What excuse were you using that situation for?

What self-image did you build as a result of that?

What was the purpose of that?

Imagine back there, that instead of using someone or something to hold yourself back as your excuse, you apologized to them, forgave them and yourself, and gave them your love. This will include you opening the gift you had for yourself as well as receiving and sharing Heaven's gift for all those present.

As it states in *A Course in Miracles*, "Attack thoughts attack my invulnerability." Become aware of judgments, criticisms and negativity that hide attacks thoughts. Give up your attack thoughts for ones of peace and reconciliation. It is in your own best interest, and in the interest of those you love, and the bonding will make your life so much easier.

Lesson 57 – The Gifts of Heaven

God is the Love that extends forever. God as a loving Father could only love us. Ideas of temptations, tests, challenges, judgment and punishments must come from our projection as they would not come from the Mind of Love. God as our Parent could only help us. This means that for every problem we have gotten ourself into, God has provided a miraculous gift to free us. These gifts exactly fit our need and the situation but because of our grievances toward, and separation from, others we will have corresponding grievances and separation from God.

When we distance ourselves from others, we cut off the grace that God is giving us. While God is Oneness and can only experience our perfection, He misses the communication from His children who have fallen into a dream of time and separation. As a result, He is always reaching out to us. Yet, the Holy Spirit, Universal Inspiration or the Tao, however you would call it, is always helping us unfold and be free, to the extent possible given our level of openness. Judgment and grievance close us to the gifts and miracles that are being given.

Let us take a two fold approach to healing our pain. First, let us ask ourselves who is the key person with whom we have grievances. If you wish a miracle then you cannot hold onto your grievance. To let go of your grievance is to help the other and yourself. They become an ally and you open to the gifts and grace of Heaven. Know that your happiness and health depend on your ability to let go of grievances. Your grievances take the place of your miracles, but you can replace grievances with miracles. Choose carefully what you want because the quality of your life depends on it. Once you have let go of the grievance in which you have invested to your detriment, and can see past the illusion about another, open yourself to receive Heaven's gift. What is that gift? Feel it. Sense it. See it. Hear it and know it. Revel in it. It is the gift of a loving Father. To give up being the prodigal child and to let go of the grievance that is causing your life to be arrested, you must be willing to make peace with whoever you are in conflict. Accept them and what has occurred, and you will be free. Forgive them, and you will be free. Let go of your grievances, and you will be free.

Recognize that this person represents self-concepts hidden inside you. How many self-concepts do you have just like this person? See these self-concepts in front of you. What do they look like? Now, melt them down to their pure energy and welcome the light and energy back inside. These self-concepts were only split off from the love inside you out of judgment, and these healing exercises free you and them. Seeing a problem in another lets you know what your hidden problem is. You would not have recognized what the problem hidden inside you was, if not for seeing it outside yourself. Pain can only come from a conflict of the self-concepts inside you. Receive Heaven's gift now and share it with the person you have projected on. Sharing the gift Heaven has for you will always increase it and help you realize that it is yours as you give it.

Lesson 58 – Pain as Authority Conflict

As I studied the mind I began to discover that all problems were a form of authority conflict, part of a power struggle. Pain is perhaps the ultimate form of authority conflict. You might begin to explore who you might be fighting with on an everyday level. Who is the significant person you are seeking to defeat? And what is this fight about? All fights show fear, a fear that you would lose something. Fear is a fantasy that something negative will occur in the future and as a result of that, some loss will also happen that must be prevented. Pain is seen as a small price to pay for preventing this supposed dire future.

The fear is an illusion and can be let go of. You no longer need to keep investing in a dire future. Let go of your belief systems that support your fear. They may support your ego, but they do not support you. Do you really want to be right about something that causes you this much pain? If your ego demands a pound of pain from you, could it really be your friend? Your ego attempts to confuse the issue by telling you it is God that wants you to suffer. This is reinforced by the book of Job in the Bible, where Job is seen as losing everything because God tested him. What is Absolute would not need to test anyone. He would know that we were created in love and innocence and remain as we were created. We could only dream it to be different than that, and we have.

The story of Christ's crucifixion is put forth as another example. "God so loved the world that He gave His only begotten Son to be tortured and crucified." But it seems to me that a loving father could not do that, much less a Divine Loving Father. There must be another way of looking at this that does not teach sacrifice as love.

Sacrifice is a psychological mistake, a form of counterfeit love. Sharing and giving always receive. Otherwise, it shows there are psychological agendas that include compensation for guilt, failure and unworthiness. Not only were the gospels changed and politicized for hundreds of years after Christ, they were changed to support the Church's authority. But even from the beginning, mistakes were made when unenlightened scribes went to interpret an enlightened being's action. All I'm saying here is that there was a mistaken emphasis put on what Christ taught, which was love and forgiveness. Neither contains sacrifice. Sabotaging Christ's message of love would be exactly what the ego would set about doing, by setting up an institution that no longer shows a way to wake up from the dream and to transcend the world and its limitations. Our collective authority conflict would manifest itself by setting up a worldly institution that taught some of the ego's vested principles along with spiritual ones.

Following this line of thinking, pain can then be seen as part of our ultimate authority conflict with God. It is a way to prove that He is not a good God at all. He wants all power for Himself and the only way for us to gain power is to kill Him, having proved by our pain that He deserves it. We seek to usurp His throne, make and interpret the world our way and do as we wish. If pain is success, then healing defeats us and must be avoided. Pain is the ultimate defiance in the most blatant form of the authority conflict. Finally, following this dire path, we die to prove that we are more powerful and that God cannot stop us. Many layers of denial go deep into the unconscious mind to hide this ultimate authority conflict and attack on Love. Healing is letting ourselves be loved and cared for. Healing is getting our life back, a little more humble and open to be shown the way. We are then a little less likely to pay a pound of pain to support our ego.

Let go of the ego payoffs that you discover are part of your authority conflict, valuing your ego over Heaven. Let go of your authority conflict, so you will stop fighting love and the great good fortune a loving Father would want to bestow on His Child.

Say the words:

I see no value in this pain.

I see no value in my purpose for pain.

I see no value in my authority conflict.

I see no value in my ego.

I would value only Love and the gifts of Love.

Lesson 59 – No Gain in Pain

We have often heard the words, "No pain, no gain." This is meant to help us 'tough out' the pain we feel as we play sports or exercise. But if we realized that there was no benefit to pain, we would give it up and healing would be immediate. To be pain free we would need to give up the hidden benefits we get from suffering. We are value-driven beings. Nothing happens to us that we do not value. We hide these choices from ourselves because they diverge from what we consciously want to believe. According to our everyday mind, we want health and strength, but pain is the evidence that we want suffering and weakness more. If we did not think they brought us something of even greater value than health and being pain free, then suffering and weakness would disappear from our lives. We must find these hidden choices for things that could never make us happy and realize there is no gain in pain. We have made a mistake and we can correct it.

Our hidden choices and values are threatened by health and strength. We seek to defend where we think our treasure is, and we foolishly believe that our hidden agenda has value. This does not make recovery easy because we have a split mind, and the mind that has the power is the one that is hidden.

Hidden values include the desire to defeat, control or possess someone, the desire for revenge, or an attempt to get a need met, or win someone from another by having them take care of us, and many others besides. In suffering, we have made a mad choice to turn pain into power and make weakness our strength.

If you were to know what it was that you were attempting to get by having pain, it's probably

If you were to know what it was that you were expecting to accomplish, it's probably

If you were to know what gain you expected to get out of pain, it's probably

Once you realize that these goals could never make you happy, you can let them go.

A *Course in Miracles* suggests a statement meant to bring immediate relief to sufferers. Simply say the words, "There is no gain at all to me in this." It states that healing occurs in exact proportion to the valuelessness that is recognized in the pain. Or to put it in other words, there is no gain in pain!

Lesson 60 – Beliefs Make the World

It is our beliefs that make the world. From our beliefs come our perception, and from our perception comes our experience. We have invested in a world of separation which is a world of pain, as pain is a consequence of separation. Beliefs are choices that we have made. The world reflects our mind and those choices have become the world we created and become embedded in. The world not only reflects what we believe, it reflects what we believe about ourselves, as every belief or concept comes from a self-concept.

Beliefs are powerful because they are backed by our mind and because we have invested in them. Everything we see and experience in the world, including pain, comes from these beliefs which are illusions. We made them up. We made them through our choice and we can let them go in the same way. It is easy to get rid of beliefs because we can change our mind about what we want to believe.

Now it is time to divest ourselves of all the beliefs we have about pain, illness and suffering. Ask yourself how many belief systems you have about pain?

Choose to let them go now.

What do you want to put in their place now?

Ask yourself how many belief systems you have about sickness.

Choose to let them go now.

What do you want to put in their place?

Ask yourself how many belief systems you have about injury.

Choose to let them go now.

What do you choose to put in their place?

Ask yourself how many belief systems you have about suffering.

Choose to let them go now.

What do you want to put in their place?

If the root of your pain is about heartbreak and betrayal, then do the same letting go exercise with them.

If the root of your pain is about guilt and failure, then do the same with your belief systems about them.

If the root of your pain is about inadequacy, loss or fear, do the same releasing exercise with them.

If it is about feeling unworthy or valueless, then do the same with these beliefs.

If it is about abandonment, feeling unwanted or rejected, then do the same with these beliefs.

Let them go and consciously choose what you want in their place.

Free your world of the beliefs in your mind.

When you have freed yourself of the significant ones regarding pain, you will be pain free.

When you release all of your beliefs, you will become enlightened because you will recognize your Self instead of all the little selves you made.

Lesson 61 – You Have Been Kidnapped by Your Ego

You have been kidnapped by your ego. We all have. Your ego is torturing you and you suffer accordingly. Your ego is not your friend. It is all that separates you from peace, love and release from pain. You may want to think twice about the price you are paying to side with your ego. You spend great effort to keep your self-image in place. You are willing to suffer so that things remain fixed, but most of all to have your sense of self with its current significance. Is this worth all the pain, when moving forward would make you less of the self you thought you were, but would also definitely make you more true to who you really are and more peaceful? This is the key to being pain free. Do you really want to pay the price of pain to keep the belief you now have about yourself?

All pain indicates that we have some buried pain in our mind, which has been displaced onto the body. You bury things because you want to maintain the status quo. You are afraid to change, yet it is change that will be your cure. But to change you have to stop protecting your ego. In the change is your release from pain.

In *A Course in Miracles*, it tells us to give our mind to the Holy Spirit and give our ego to Christ. So today, if you are willing, give your ego into the hands of Christ and ask for the change that Heaven wants to give you. It would be one step closer to the peace and joy that are characteristics of Heaven. Allow anything that got you into your present predicament, and which you need to let go of, to come to your mind so that you can understand the mistake you made. Let your desire to see bring about the natural breakthrough such awareness brings. You no longer have to keep a certain self-image. Whatever mistake you made is rendered innocent, transforming into freedom the guilt which the ego has made. The guilt is a root cause of your pain, which your ego led you to bury and deny. Let this be your day to birth yourself to a newer, truer you.

Heaven is behind you, and all the world will benefit from another layer of separation removed. And remember anything you don't like about yourself is simply a self-concept.

Accept it, and it's released. Own it, and it's integrated into a new wholeness. Let it go, and you no longer have to go around supporting an expensive self-image that you have to pay for with pain.

Lesson 62 – Freeing the World of Pain

"What keeps the world in chains but your beliefs?

And what can save the world except your Self?"

A Course in Miracles

As we realize that perception is not something imposed - it is decided - we become empowered. The decisions we have already made have become our beliefs about the world. As such, they are unreflected on. We think that this is the way the world is, because we experience it that way and almost everyone agrees with us, not realizing that the experiences we have of the world are as we decided. The world of our perception and our beliefs support each other. The fact is everyone sees a different world, some much brighter than others. In general, we agree consensually on the construction of reality. But physicists, some mystics, the enlightened, and *A Course in Miracles* agree that we have imposed our own choices about how the world is on the waves and particles of light.

A Course in Miracles puts it thus:

There is no world. Healing is the gift and you can lose

it from all the things you ever thought it was

by merely changing all the thoughts that gave

it these appearances. The sick are healed as you

let go thoughts of sickness and the dead arise when

you let thoughts of life replace all thoughts

ever held of death.

To free your mind of every kind of pain is but to

change your mind about yourself. Release the

world! Release your mind and you will look upon a

world released.

As we give up all of our belief systems and self-concepts, the mind clears and we become more and more conflict free. All our beliefs are actually beliefs about ourselves. Typically, we tend to clear the negative self-concepts by letting go, self-forgiveness, acceptance and integration. This generates new wholeness. We hide the dark self-concepts from ourselves because we are afraid of the guilt and self-hatred, which is vast within us, but buried and compensated for. So, if we have the courage to face our shadow figures, negativity, guilt, feelings of failure and valuelessness, we can effectively move toward wholeness. Once we have exchanged the negative self-concepts for wholeness then we can begin to ferret out even the positive self-concepts to replace them with greater wholeness and light.

Changing our mind by healing our belief systems is a tried and true method, as we have beliefs about everything and everyone. We have already mentioned that to experience pain we must have beliefs about pain, suffering, injury, victims, villains, fear, guilt, revenge, holding on, etc. But we also have other psychological beliefs that tell a story about what happened to us that got us into our present position. It would have been a heartbreak, betrayal, abandonment, abuse or some interesting story that would be filled with beliefs and judgments.

Yet, besides healing all of our self-concepts, step by step, there is also a quicker way, which is to recognize ourself as spirit. This lifts us from the self we are so obsessed about to recognition of our Oneness with God.

"Ideas leave not their source," as *A Course in Miracles* states. We did not leave God. Spirit created us spirit and we are still in Oneness. We are one Self in spite of our present dream and beliefs, pain and separation. The recognition of ourself as spirit puts the body into balance. It frees us of the conflicts of the mind that we displace onto the body. It restores us to our one true identity that will be made clear once we have removed all of our self-concepts. As we take the healing path and jettison the belief systems that are cheating us of the joy that comes of joining, it becomes easier to remember we are spirit. Yet, some people can leap forward in life and save themselves untold amounts of time and pain. There are others that see we are spirit when they are at the point of death and as a result come back restored spiritually and physically.

Follow whichever path of realization calls to you. Even if you take the step-by-step path of healing your negative self-concepts and then your positive ones, so that there will always be less of you and more of Heaven, it is important *to plant the seed of recognizing that you are spirit, one with God, a part of all creation, filled with love and light.*

Spend some time meditating on these thoughts today because they bring freedom from pain and release from suffering.

Lesson 63 – The Heart of the Matter

There is a story you are telling about how you got to this point. It tells what happened to you, that you would somehow end up suffering as you are. This story leads up to the present point, but where did it begin and who did it begin with? What happened to you that you are in such a sorry state?! We don't end up in such a state without blaming someone else for us ending up where we are. What happened to you? What is your story? How did you come to be here in this situation? Tell yourself the story. Write it out. Tape it or tell it to a friend. You have probably been telling it to yourself over and over again, and probably to anyone else who would listen. What is your story? How did you come to be the way you are?

What kind of story is it? Are you the hero, the victim, the villain or all of these three parts? Was there a stupid mistake, a fatal flaw that led to your downfall, or was it a betrayal or profound disappointment that got you here?

Examine this story. Reflect on this story. It will contain many of the belief systems that are haunting you. Is it worth the story to pay the price of pain? Do you notice that now it supports your ego rather than you? Do you notice your story is all about you, to the point of being self-obsessed? A story that is all about you, no matter what the story is, will be a story of suffering. Besides all the secondary benefits of having such a story, the main reason is to support our ego and our sense of separation. This is not in our own best interest, nor that of those around us. Who did you need to make a bad guy so that you could go independent? Have you blocked all of their love for you since that time? You could realize that it is just a story you made up to glorify yourself, even if it is all dark glamour, and let the love in instead. You don't have to glorify your self when glory is a key attribute of your Self. But your little self feels deprived and so tries to give itself significance and attention. You could have peace instead of this. You could have love and bonding instead of this story. The brilliance that would shine out of you, as you gave up this story, would more than make up for the clamor for attention and sympathy of the ego's story that you have invested in. Your story is one of deprivation, either in the story line itself or by the fact that it is a story.

131

To reach Wholeness we will have given up both our negative and our positive stories. See what you are using your story for, and then let your story go. Let Heaven rewrite the story for you in loving gentleness. If you look at the story, you will notice that it was just an excuse to hide your fear of love. Letting go of this story is one giant step in letting the love in.

Let yourself be loved today. Especially open the door that was closed to love when your story began. Let all that love in. It will be a giant step in releasing your pain. Make that choice with Heaven. It will be a giant step back toward your Self, the Self you share with everyone.

Lesson 64 – Pain is Inevitable

There is a saying in Buddhism:

Pain is inevitable

but suffering is optional.

Having bodies and experiencing ourselves as separate means that we will experience pain. Yet, we can experience it and not suffer because of it. To experience pain courageously is the most basic of the healing methods. We simply experience what is there without running from it. There is a certain quotient of pain we have all come to heal in our lives. Some of it is existential. These are the issues that we are heir to, as the result of living in a body in the world. These include experiences such as pain, age and death. Existential pain can also come from suffering meaninglessness and questioning why we are here. Existential pain includes valuelessness because if there is no meaning, there is no value. If avoided, this becomes psychological suffering and, if we avoid our psychological-emotional pain, then we displace it onto our body.

Pain can get spread between the existential, psychological and physical. When it becomes a vicious circle of these elements, the pain is continuous with each one adding to the other. But we can wade into our suffering and, simply by feeling the existential and psychological pain, we can diminish our suffering in general. As we witness the pain we are in and pay close attention to it, it not only unfolds into a flow, it also begins to diminish.

One tradition states that Christ never suffered on the cross, contrary to Mel Gibson's movie *The Passion of the Christ*. Jesus had forgiven so completely that he was the best example of his own teachings of love and forgiveness. He not only loved his enemies, He also did not experience them as enemies. He simply saw them as not knowing what they were doing, "Father, forgive them; for they know not what they do." This lets us know the power of healing and gives us hope about freeing ourselves, not only from suffering, but also from pain.

If you try to avoid the suffering that you are in, you not only delay the inevitable, you build it up inside you. But if you face it, you can move through it. We usually do anything in our power to avoid both pain and suffering. While I am not simply advocating suffering in pain, I am advocating not avoiding your pain. Avoidance can only build it up to be faced later. Though there are exercises in this book that suggest you aggressively feel the very physicality of your pain, most exercises are about transforming the emotional pain so that the roots of the physical pain are removed.

If you are planning to face your suffering, first simply witness it, then exaggerate it. You can take control of the pain by increasing it. Once in control, you can lessen the pain more easily. Make yourself into a bullet and fly through the suffering; it will lessen your pain. Take the right attitude toward your pain and it will build compassion and wisdom. But if you use your pain for some special agenda or payoff, you will suffer from it and because of it, and it will continue.

Physical pain is there to let us know something is wrong; it is like having our finger in a flame. Emotional pain is also an indicator of a mistake. It lets us know we are sticking our finger in an emotional fire that is not only unnecessary, it is also a mistake. As we free ourselves of emotional pain, we can face the existential pain and diminish physical pain. If we solve the mystery of the meaning of the pain, and witness this bottom-line, it brings freedom from pain. Spirituality, and recognizing ourselves as spirit, is the antidote to existential pain. Even meaninglessness is easily resolved if you would ask Heaven, "What is my meaning?" Heaven and Spirit are the essence of meaning itself because it is love.

The mind is the doctor of the body. It is the mind that heals us. As you hear the words that come through, you will experience the grace the words reflect. You will only **not** hear the words if you are afraid to hear them, afraid of change or you are fighting Heaven. This means you are in an authority conflict and supplanting Heaven's meaning with your own. Good Luck with that! That's a sure fire way to experience a good deal of pain.

So I would like to change the saying from, "Pain is inevitable but suffering is optional," to:

Pain is normal in this human world,

but in the long run unnecessary.

Suffering meanwhile comes

of siding with the ego for something

we value more than peace.

Let us value peace instead.

Lesson 65 – Wishing the World Away

"There is no world apart from what you wish, and herein lies your ultimate release. Change your mind on what accordingly.

Ideas leave not their source."

A Course in Miracles

Besides our beliefs, wishing, choosing and desiring the world to be the way it is, are the other major ways that we make the world around us. We want to see things a certain way. We are curious about what would happen if a certain thing occurred. We want to have an experience of something. This can all make the world.

We hide the fact that we do this. We can choose something in one second and repress it in the next, or even make the choice subconsciously. This choosing, that makes our reality, corroborates the findings in Quantum Physics about the nature of reality as we experience it. If we begin to dwell on this, and what it means in terms of pain, it opens up new levels of understanding. We wished for the pain; we wished for the story that led to the pain. Of course, this is not what our conscious mind is telling us, but not only is that the smallest part of the mind, it is also the part that felt we couldn't deal with the truth and so denied and buried it. Our lack of courage to face mistaken motivation and idle wishes led us to make a subconscious mind and thus not take responsibility for what happens to us. This may be the biggest trap of all.

So **let's pretend** you wanted the pain and your life as you experience it. Pretending helps you see what you have hidden from yourself. Why would you want it to be that way? Now we know you really don't want pain or victim situations but that is just the denial of the conscious mind on one hand, which causes us to push things into our mind that we then dissociate and repress, and what is in your deepest mind on the other. Obviously you are experiencing pain. This means that there are clearly both subconscious and unconscious patterns that have more power. So let's pretend you wanted your situation exactly as it came down. How come?

One of the first principles I learned about the subconscious was that "intentions equal results." In other words, what happens is exactly what you want to have happen. As you see your intentions, you get to make another choice, one in which you could not only see a better, pain free world, but also see a world completely different to the one you made. You could rechoose after you found your hidden payoffs. What were they? The fear of love, the desire to be independent and separate, the need for attention and significance are just a few of the many motivations that might show themselves.

Once you see what your motivations are, and examine them with your conscious mind, you can see that they were a really bad deal and choose again. Another exercise is to meditate on the world in front of you. Realize it is just illusory. It is your waking dream that is generated through wish fulfillment, as all dreams are. Now you can will to see beyond this world, to one full of light and love that you are a part of. Imagine that this dream world was a stage, and you could walk behind the scenery and the stage itself, and come to the door behind the stage. The play on the stage has been so distracting that you never thought to come here before. Now open that door to the light that is filled with joy. Know the real world is made of love and you are part of it.

Lesson 66 – Pain as Fear of Responsibility

Responsibility is a powerful trait and it is simple in that responsibility is a response to what is needed. By responding, we generate bonding and bonding creates positive flow. Denial of responsibility puts us in the weakest of positions. We are at the effect of outside agents and as a result, anything can happen. When we choose to see the body as that which made us sick because of outside agents, such as bacteria, germs, viruses, etc. then we have little or no power and it reinforces the idea of us as a body. If we see our body as our identity, then we see ourself as a body on the way to death.

I would like to propose a healing alternative that categorically wins back responsibility. To realize one's responsibility we must recognize that our illness and pain come from mistaken decisions that we have made. This would change our whole perception of ourself and the world. It would also mean that responsibility lies in our hands. As a result, medicines and procedures that work simply reflect our own positive choices. What works as an outside agent simply shows our own inner desires, measured against our hidden self-attack. Whichever is the stronger will be shown by the outcome. With this outlook, we would realize that the world does nothing to us that we did not want it to do.

Pain represents faulty problem solving on our part, which we then relegate to the subconscious and experience ourself as the victim of our world. It means that we saw something more threatening than sickness and pain. We decided how we would deal with the threat, and then set up defense after defense, including illness, to counter the threat that we believed was real. But then we have to repress the fact that we were the one who decided these things, and forget that we forgot it. This makes it look as if something outside us is affecting us against our will. We have disowned what happened to us, thinking that it is happening to us by 'natural' means. Nothing could be more unnatural but, having convinced ourselves collectively of this, we blithely live in a world full of victims who have not taken responsibility for what occurs. More and more is pressed into the subconscious, as we take less and less accountability for what is occurring in our lives until, disappointed, we finally go down the path to death, cursing ourself, life, God and those whose fault we think it was.

To take responsibility allows us to see the sick and mistaken choices we made. And having seen the futility of such painful, untrue choices, we would naturally make another choice to give them up.

Let us now take responsibility, not only for the pain we suffer now, but for **all the times** in our life that we suffered.

- What fear were we trying to avoid by having such suffering?

- What was it we were trying to gain by having suffering in our life then and now?

- Who were we trying to control by our suffering, proving we should be in charge?

- How were we trying to control ourselves by what happened?

Seeing these answers, and whatever else comes to mind, would allow us to see what we fail to gain by such unreasonable choices and we would make other, truer choices. Commit to responsibility today. Commit to winning back your mind. Commit to seeing what has been denied so it can be released. Win your mind back so it is used for joy instead of pain.

Lesson 67 – Pain – The Ultimate Authority Conflict

Now it is time to present pain in a new light, one that we have hidden in the deepest depths of the unconscious because we would not like to see ourselves in this way at all. As a matter of fact, it is hard for most of us to believe that it is so. When I first read these core dynamics in *A Course in Miracles*, in regard to how we use pain as part of our authority conflict with God, to prove He is a bad God and we should be put in His place, I could see the truth of it. Later, I could feel the truth of it and, about twenty years ago with a few gifted clients, was able to penetrate to that level of the mind for the resolution of such impacted problems. Once we examine this issue with the light of reason, we realize that such buried reasoning is foolish, and is actually no real reason at all. In this way, we are willing to give up that mistaken purpose that we have been willing to pay the price of pain for.

Now if we are responsible for our pain, then obviously the reasoning and intention behind it must be madness. And this dynamic of pain *at the deepest level of the mind*, reflects our hidden penchant for stealing power, God's power, as we seek to usurp His throne and place ourself on it. We project that God is mad, power hungry, hoarding all authority and command. As such then, the only way to thwart God and prove we are more powerful than Him, is to die. This demonstrates, at least to ourselves, that we are more powerful because we can die and God cannot stop us. In the context of this insane reasoning where we have turned God into something other than a loving Father through our own crazy projections, the path of healing becomes a path of sanity in which we take responsibility for our thoughts because they cause our experience.

If this is so, then healing would then also reflect where we have lost, and God has triumphed over us. This way of thinking is what we must hide from ourselves at all costs. When pain has become a way of winning, then we have made weakness our strength. In ultimate rebellion and defiance, we turn away from grace and prove what a sad, hopeless and helpless creature we are. In choosing death ourselves, death then shows our strength, because instead of being killed by God, who we see as the Great Enemy, we steal His power and do it ourselves.

Do not hide this from yourself. Look at this dynamic clearly. Even if you don't believe it, examine it. Once you see it, you will naturally realize the foolish mistake it is. So, of course, it is repressed and denied. We typically all have a similar pattern going on with our parents, as a dynamic of the Oedipal Conspiracy. We have projected murderous thoughts on to the parent of the same sex. In the attempt to steal the opposite sex parent, we come to believe we are failures, thieves, murderers and betrayers. While these shadow figures, which are repressed, wouldn't stand the light of reason in our conscious mind, we still believe these things about ourselves and punish ourselves accordingly.

We bury such dynamics by compensating and being good, nice, deeply religious people. Having judged the power-monger within us and thus strengthened it, then we must bury it. Hiding from ourselves what we really are makes us the proverbial 'divided house' and, as the Biblical saying goes, "A house divided against itself shall not stand."

We have buried what is in conflict with our conscious mind, but it is no less a conflict. The authority conflict generates fear and pain. We are afraid to acknowledge the part of our ego mind that is a 'sick puppy', paying the price of pain to hide our desperate desire to be the 'Boss' and control everything.

It is time to see what is there and let go of such insanity. Let God be God, and let us return to being His child.

Lesson 68 – Pain as Level Confusion

There are three parts to us and ultimately only one is true. The first and most basic is the body. Most people have identified themselves as a body. As such, things happen to 'us' that are out of our control and that we must suffer with. The second aspect of ourselves is our mind, or soul if you wish. It is the conflicts of the mind, visited on the body, that lead to sickness and pain. You could imagine from this level that your body is a poor dumb animal that you beat when you get upset at yourself, your work, relationships or life.

When I first began working in holistic health, I found direct connection between health and healing the past. The first client I worked with at a holistic level, received spiritual healing, therapy from me and changed the course of her nutrition. I worked with her through her early childhood trauma of physical torture and the later mental and emotional torture by her late husband. Six months after she had originally been diagnosed she met the doctor who had referred her to a specialist. She had been so sick when he had first seen her that he blurted out, "What are you doing still alive?"

My friend who had had three major tumors, one the size of a rugby ball, tried to tell him what she had done to help herself, but he went on, "No, no, never mind. Just keep doing it."

This was my first hands on experience in which I saw the mind-body connection. Much later, I learned that the mind and the body are not connected as such, except when there is level confusion. One way to achieve health is to see them as completely separate, so we don't make the body a 'whipping boy' for the mind. This is level confusion at its worst.

The third level, which puts everything right, is ourself as spirit. Evolution could be said to be the gradual realization of the mind that it is spirit. This takes us out of time and into timelessness. There are three distinct levels and the higher the level of realization, namely of spirit, the more unlimited we are.

To identify and realize ourselves as spirit is to heal automatically. To separate the mind from the body is to realize that the conflicts of the mind have no effect at all on the body, because the conflicts don't leave the mind *unless we have level confusion*. If things don't truly leave the mind, then they have no effect on the body. This realization also heals the body.

To identify ourselves as a body is then a defense, a part of our authority conflict against the Creator who created us as spirit. Like comes from like. So from God, the Spirit of Oneness, we were created as spirit. From Love, we were created as love. From Light, we were created as light. But in our mad dream of separation, which is also a dream of suffering, we rebelled to build a physical world. We may dream we live here but it is not our home, and we will eventually reach our Home that is even now calling us back to ourself as spirit, a part of All That Is.

Let us realize our body is our vehicle to learn, grow and share. Love and healing move us inexorably toward the joy of Oneness. We were created as part of this Oneness. And while we are still in a body and using our mind, let us not take out our conflicts on the body. Today let us know ourselves as spirit, with all the love and peace that no longer allow us to defend against the truth of ourselves as spirit. This brings light where there was darkness, and releases us from pain and limitation.

Lesson 69 – Personalizing Pain

One of the ways to generate pain or increase it, is to personalize it. I recently worked with a woman whose daughter and grandchildren had come to visit her. She made a really big deal of the visit, rented a baby elephant, cleaned up her house in a major way, and had many treats and activities lined up, including meeting the staff at her business.

The woman telling me this story was crying her heart out. "My daughter doesn't love me. She stayed one night, and then moved herself and my grandchildren to a five star hotel."

I said to her, "It's OK. Your daughter loves you. She wanted to stay with her new boyfriend and his children who were at the five star hotel. You don't have air-conditioning and it's the hottest part of the summer. Your daughter is just self-centered. She's doing what she wants to do. It's not personal."

The woman understood immediately, and felt relieved. I also pointed out that her daughter's behavior was similar to how the woman's own mother had acted toward her, which also wasn't personal. It was just her mother's way of doing things. I noted that if the mother and daughter were like this, there was obviously some lesson she was to learn. The first lesson was that what was hurting was a need she was trying to get her daughter, and previously her mother, to meet. When a need is involved, there is a kind of taking and any form of taking is eventually unsuccessful and leads to feeling hurt or defeated.

Many times people with physical pain personalize it, also asking, "Why is this happening to me? Why is God doing this to me? How come things like this always happen to me?"

This is a mistake. It's not personal. It is the same with the emotional events that led to the physical pain.

Many people are suffering many kinds of pain, right this very minute. Pain goes on all the time. It is not just about you. If you get over yourself, you will see that people act in hurtful ways because the dissociated pain inside them leads them to do things for themselves, either to medicate the pain or to take care of some need.

Pain is happening to many others right now. Bless them and bless yourself. You are not alone or unique in this experience. Have compassion for yourself and others, and please don't increase your pain by personalizing it. As you realize that many others are in a similar situation, your heart will flower, your compassion will grow and it will lessen your pain.

Lesson 70 – Your Attention

Pain is very distracting. It has us remove our attention from the conflict within ourselves that led to the pain, and puts it on the pain itself. Even then, we do not fully pay attention to the pain because if we put our total attention on the pain, it would begin to unfold. Physical pain, when deeply witnessed, begins to shift so that the sensation of the suffering changes as it is truly experienced. At first the pain might possibly get worse because we have been trying to suppress the suffering and toughing it out rather than feeling it. But whether that is the case or not, if we witness our suffering, at some point, it begins to unfold, sensation by sensation, and untangle itself. As this occurs, we can handle it so much better.

With emotional pain, if we freely give ourselves to paying attention to it, it begins to show us the issue surrounding and driving it. The root of this emotional charge is from the past. When we witness our suffering and don't turn away from it, it eventually takes us back to the roots where it began and, if we continue to watch it closely, even the roots will untangle. Of course, the final root is the original separation or fall from Heaven. This is the primordial guilt, separation and pain that feeds all the collective, unconscious and subconscious patterns that are painfully in the way of our witnessing and healing the original separation.

So many times when we are in pain, we run away from it with drugs, entertainment, etc. This just puts off the inevitable. The pain will wait for us or seek some other form. So many times, instead of witnessing our suffering, we watch our 'self' suffer so that the experience of pain becomes the experience of the self suffering. This is a crucial difference as the latter builds the ego, which sooner or later brings more suffering, while to simply witness it leads to its healing. It is a difference of witnessing the suffering we are experiencing, or to witness the suffering **we** are experiencing as a way of being special.

So today do not be afraid of your suffering. It will only increase if you resist it. Your fear increases your pain. Do not turn away from your pain, turn into it. If you are in very intense pain, then you may need something to lessen the pain enough even to do this exercise. Take responsibility for your healing and choose what is best for you. The key is to turn in the direction of the pain rather than away from it. Pay attention to it. Let it teach you. Let your heart flower in compassion as you realize how much of the world suffers along with you. Notice when you turn away from your pain, you witness **you** experiencing the suffering rather than witnessing the suffering itself. This will only build your ego and you will use it to tell *your* story. Your separation is the very heart of your pain. Simply pay attention to your suffering, and what separates you from yourself, the light within, others, and the Divine. You will begin to unfold toward joining once more.

Lesson 71 – Enslaving the Body

To enslave the body is to make it endure all the whims of our thoughts, conflicts and emotions. The body is tortured for the problems and lack that is in our mind. Imagine we had a pet cat or dog that we treated as cruelly as our body. We would probably be arrested. The fact that we are taking a problem out on our body means that, someplace within our mind, we are in conflict and thus arrested mentally and emotionally. When this is displaced physically onto our body, it is a sign that we do not wish to deal with it or that the conflict is coming from deep in the mind, covered over by denial, dissociation and now distraction. When we attempt to enslave our body or another person, for that matter, it is a compensation for the feelings of helplessness, lack of self-worth and enslavement within. The body is, in fact, neutral and will continue to support us in its function as a vehicle for learning and healing. It is like our token in a board game or our figure in a video game.

In 1983, I heard Dr. David Bohm, a leading Quantum Physicist, state that in quantum physics they had just discovered that we are not really here, that our bodies are a three dimensional projected hologram, and that they were now attempting to discover who was projecting us. This is the same as if we were playing a video game and we became so identified with the game that we lost sight of who we were, and thought we were the character in the game. It is like watching a movie so intensely we forget it's a movie.

We think we are our body and not the consciousness that drives it. As we evolve further, we will discover that we are not our consciousness but the spirit it has covered. Consciousness exists in dualism, separation and conflict. Consciousness is always consciousness of an object that we experience as outside us, separate from us. Awareness on the other hand comes from the realm of spirit, it is what exists in Oneness.

If we learn to distinguish the three levels of body, mind and spirit, we would learn to separate them and not misuse them. We can identify with any of the three. We can think that we are our bodies and suffer the weakness, insecurity and victimization that identifying with the body brings about. Or we can think we are our consciousness. Our mind then directs our activity, forward movement, and healing. Recognizing we are our mind, we would more naturally take responsibility for the state of our lives and the condition of our body as a learning vehicle. But the highest identification is with our spirit. This would put the other two levels into balance. It would heal the conflicts of the mind as well as the dysfunctions of the body. It would open us to grace and Divine Love.

When I had my near death experience, I left my body and it felt as if I was a world away from my body. I floated down the first corridor, feeling entirely conscious, peaceful and aware as the senses of my body were shutting down. I saw how easy death was. It was like falling asleep. Yet when I came to the abyss at the end of the first corridor, I decided not to 'give up,' turned around and floated back up the corridor, making the jump back into my body, which was in a good bit of pain.

At that point, I realized I was not my body but my soul. If I had gone down the second corridor, as Dr. Elizabeth Kubler-Ross later explained to me, I would have seen the light and probably had the realization of myself as light or spirit.

We do not need such dramatic experiences to realize that we are not our body. To realize we are a consciousness gives us great power. To realize we are spirit is to realize even greater power and our Oneness. When we are one with God as Spirit, we are unlimited. There is nothing we cannot do and the power of miracles is ours.

Today, realize yourself as the one playing the video game, and not the character that's inside, acting it out. Ask your spirit for the inspiration, guidance and grace that would remove the fear that keeps you using the body to distract and delay you from the lesson and healing in front of you. This lesson will always be one that dissolves fear, heals guilt and releases the pain.

Ask for your lesson regarding pain to be easily learned, and the fear and guilt which made the pain be quickly dispersed, so that you are naturally moved forward to the next step in progress, power and wholeness.

Lesson 72 – How You Got to Where You Are

We are story tellers and myth makers. We are a legend in our own mind. We tell stories about everything. It is how our minds work. This would be a good time for you to write, record or tell a willing friend how you got to be in the pain you are in. Embellish your story. Exaggerate it. Begin the story as far back as you can go. Tell what happened to you, that a good person like you became the home of pain. Prepare whatever medium you will use to tell your story. Reflect for just a minute and then begin. Take as long as you want but do not draw it out so long that you lose the point. If you have artistic ability then make pictures of the most salient points. Do not use your judgment in your pictures. Let them paint or draw you. There is another purpose to the pictures which has to do with healing, rather than art.

Once you have written, recorded or told your story, read it, play it back or listen to a friend recounting the highlights. Examine the drawings if any. What do you notice when you reflect on the story and paintings.

Next, ask yourself how many stories like this one you have inside

Ask yourself the effect of these stories on your life

Ask yourself what purpose this story serves for you

What was it you were trying *to get* by telling this story?

What did it allow you to do?

What excuse did you get to have by telling this story of pain?

How, and for what purpose have you used your story and its incipient pain?

After you have finished answering these questions, reflect on whether you succeeded or not in your attempt to get what you wanted? Ask yourself if this story and the pain made you happy, because both were an attempt to get something that you thought would make you happier?

Did it work?

At the deepest levels, every story is an attempt to give us a stronger ego. Your ego is what separates you from others, life and success. Do you really want to build your ego at the expense of your health and your life?

Often, your stories go back to the fundamental patterns that are directing your life. Notice what effect this fundamental pattern has had on your life. Reflect on it. Witness it. Study it.

When you have *fully paid attention to the pattern,* it will spontaneously change, especially after you realize your hidden agenda. You won't even have to decide about it or let it go. The story will unfold in a positive manner. It will do what occurs next in its unfolding and, as it changes, you will find new freedom. Keep paying attention to it until it has completely unfolded in a positive way. If it seems to be stuck, ask yourself what you are afraid to let go of. Let it go and continue.

Lesson 73 – Blessing the Pain Away

Blessing is the opposite of judgment and as *A Course in Miracles* states, "From judgment comes all the suffering of the world." Blessing is built on acceptance, and it adds an aspect of giving on our part, to which Heaven adds a portion of grace. Blessing generates flow.

Today begin by blessing your pain. Bless it frequently. Bless yourself and every single person you come in contact with today. Bless your room, your bed, your meals. Partner with Heaven in giving your blessings today, such as a "God bless you."

Bless your day before you begin. Bless it once more when you have finished. Bless your sleep. Bless your family, both living and deceased. Bless your friends. Bless your partner. Bless the sun. Bless nature. Bless the rain. Bless the moon and stars. Bless your car, your house, your clothes and your work. Bless life and bless your life. Bless God and bless your next step. Bless sex, intimacy, your work and your family. Bless your enemies. Bless your money, health and your work.

Never stop blessing. Bless with a glad heart. Bless all those you cursed consciously or unconsciously. Bless everyone and everything today. Bless unceasingly because blessings like trust unfold things in a positive way. Today let blessing move you forward. Bless your body. Bless your mind and bless your circumstances. People need blessing most when their situations are at their worst.

Let blessing become a way of life for you, especially when you are tempted to judge. Judgment makes you right, and locks you into the situation as you have judged it. Bless instead. Blessing makes a positive contribution toward a person or situation that was in need of help.

Lesson 74 – Release from Pain

Release from pain is easy if you are willing to change your mind. There is some place inside you where you are in conflict. Belief systems are caroming off each other, or you are enslaved to beliefs of guilt, pain, or self-expectations. Your ego has convinced you the future will be even more painful than the present. You will be forced to endure something as bad as the worst survival situations of your past.

Actually, that is most likely what you are enduring now. The pain of past survival situations is feeding their pain into this present situation. The emotional charge of the past is bleeding into the present situation. On the other hand, your willingness to take responsibility for the past and the present allows you to change your mind, first about yourself and then about all that is causing your pain. If you are suffering, there is something you haven't let yourself off the hook for as yet. You are suffering where you haven't let others off the hook. Your judgment and grievances hide your deeper guilt. Your grievances come because people did not act according to the scripts that you, as the leading actor, assigned them at a subconscious level. But at an even deeper level of the unconscious, people acted exactly as you wanted them to act. At the unconscious level, everyone and everything in your world is acting out your wishes. They are playing the scripts and telling the stories that come from the interaction of your myriad self-concepts. Everyone is acting out how you used to be or how you believe you are. That you are suffering so acutely speaks of certain survival situations of the past that are feeding into the present.

These events may still be repressed, or you may be aware of them but as yet haven't fully gotten all the suffering or emotional charge off them. You have not gone through the birth that would free you by facing all the pain you avoided from your past. When you don't finish a situation through emotional birth, you keep it as an ego agenda of unfinished business which keeps coming up, time and again, until it is finished.

How are you now using that situation from the past? Can you take full responsibility for it, so as to move through it all the quicker? Was the situation set up to get something, protect a certain fear, hide, run from your purpose, rebel, have an excuse, hold onto or have an indulgence, be right about your beliefs, gain control *or, bottom line, build your "self" by siding with your ego?* This last is the core dynamic of all survival situations.

In rare cases, people in the healing profession have actively chosen, at a soul level even before they have come into this life, to throw themselves into a place of pain to learn, lead or direct them to the healing path. There is an ancient prayer which I believe comes from Tibetan Buddhism which goes:

Please, lead me into all misfortune.

For only by that path can I transform

what is negative into the positive.

If this is your deepest intention, then I wish you all the courage to face your suffering so that you turn your pain into birthing of a new, more essential self that has the power to transform your and others' present misfortune.

Ask to see the root causes of your suffering. Go through the suffering. Let your Guardian Angel help and hold you through this root experience. See the reliving of it as a birth situation, look at it with new eyes. Declare everyone's innocence. Keep to the feeling. Burn through the pain until you are at peace. Give the soul level gifts you have come to give to the people in those situations, but do so even before the painful events occur so that you obviate them. Receive and give Heaven's gift to everyone in the situation. At one level, you inherited the pain they were feeling inside. But healing them and yourself at an unconscious level, you have created a shortcut through your suffering.

Lesson 75 – You are Spirit

This is the answer to all your problems regarding pain. By recognizing yourself as spirit, the mind quietens and becomes conflict free. The body becomes the neutral, healthy vehicle it was meant to be. The body can be healed, as the mind which is identifying with it rids itself of conflict. This is the healing of "level-confusion", as *A Course in Miracles* calls it. Many people don't even recognize that they have a spirit. They live a life of seeking reward and pleasure, not realizing that the higher reaches of pleasure come from joy, which is a derivative of love and sharing.

If we remove our identification from the body and the mind through recognition of truth that we are spirit, there can be immediate results. Otherwise, if not immediate results, we can move in this direction through choice and then through will. The recognition of ourself as spirit brings peace to the mind and balances the body. Spirit is the most essential part of us. All the rest will pass. The body will fade, the soul-mind will evolve until we recognize ourselves as spirit. This recognition of ourselves as spirit will save us from 'doing time,' help us realize that we cannot be harmed, because we are safe. There is nothing we need, because we are whole. There is no conflict, because we are healed. As spirit, we recognize our Oneness. Where there is Oneness there is no suffering.

We have spent a lifetime building a self and we are highly invested in it. This gives us an identity in the world vis-a-vis others. When we recognize ourselves as spirit then we move beyond valuing the world and trying to get something from it. As spirit, we have everything and we are everything, because we are in the Mind of God as His creation.

The self we have built up began at about the age of one and a half. It was meant to fade away at eighteen or nineteen years of age, so that our connection with the richness of nature, and with others, ourself and the Divine, would lead to the ease, joy and success that comes of such connection. But somehow the ego fought for its existence and never let go of its identity. It is still fighting for it. Bottom line, it is our self that is suffering, a so-called 'innocent victim' of someone or something acting badly. This gives us the right to justifiable anger, which is an attempt to displace the guilt we felt at the separation or "the Fall" into the dream of separation. This is the primordial conflict from which all conflict arises, and we are still caught until we recognize the fallacy of the separation, and that what was whole as Spirit could not be separated. We could only dream that we separated because what is true cannot be lost. Now is the time to begin our awakening to who we really are.

Let this day be a commitment to wholeness, a commitment to the light and love that we are as spirit. Let us bring that recognition into our day and any time something disturbs our peace, whether it be emotional or physical, repeat the words,

"As a child of God I am spirit. I choose the truth of this reality now."

Lesson 76 – To Rest in God

Today, let yourself rest in God.

Let all your worries be given to God.

Let your future be given to God.

Let your past and all its mistakes be given to God for correction. No need to defend yourself today; it only calls in attack.

Let God be in charge of you today. You can rest easy today, knowing your back is covered.

Let all of your jobs today be God's jobs.

Let everything be accomplished through you today, but not by you.

Live in grace today.

Live in the Love that is God's.

Let all of your needs be met by this Love. God being Love has no Will for you to suffer. If it is not God's Will, it is not your true will.

Rest in God today.

Let His angels minister to you.

Take the load off your shoulders and off your mind today.

Rest in God. You are His child.

Rest easy in His Arms today.

Release the heaviness from your heart. You are beloved of God Himself.

Give up all sacrifice and martyrdom. You no longer need to do this to save anyone or to hide your fear of all the good things that await you.

Rest in God today.

Lesson 77 – Christ's Promise

Just before Christ left the Earth, he made a promise to us. He promised that he would not leave us comfortless. He did not promise this to Christians only. There were no Christians at this point. He made the promise to all of us. When we are suffering pain, whether physical, emotional or mental, it would be wise of us to take these words to heart.

Comfort is around us spiritually if we are open to it. If we need comfort in the way of a person, he or she will be there. If we need comfort in a certain path of healing, it will be there. If we need a certain remedy, it will be there. All that it takes on our part is to avail ourselves of it. If we are not open to it, it does not matter how good it is. Thoreau wrote, "Only that day dawns to which we are awake." So let us be awake to receive what is there to provide comfort for us. Thoreau finished by stating: "And the light that is too bright blinds us." This is not really about the light but about our ability to receive it. Heaven's answer to our suffering is a miracle but we are afraid of it. If it threatened our belief systems then we would be too afraid, as we value "our way" more than the way out. Let us ask for the courage and the dissolution of our fear that we might receive the answer, along with the comfort we need. Let us accept Christ's promise. Let us allow our need to be filled.

The Holy Spirit has been called the Comforter. This is that aspect of God that knows exactly what we need on the Earth, as we need it. The Holy Spirit is the Voice for God, giving us the guidance that we need to get out of every difficulty, and to find the way Home. The Holy Spirit is the bringer of miracles. Let them be brought. Give your fear to the Holy Spirit so that this pain, which is a distraction to keep us from taking the next step forward, melts away and the next step is brought to you in a beautiful flow.

Don't let yourself be comfortless when you have been promised comfort. Open yourself to receive and wait with expectancy. If you are suffering, what comes to you can be better than Christmas. Have the same joyful expectancy as you did when you were a small child waiting for Christmas morning.

Lesson 78 – Be Not Afraid

The phrase most often used in the Bible is ="Be not afraid." These are words to take to heart. There is no problem that does not hide fear. There is no pain that does not hide fear. But if God created us in His own image, then we are spirit and as spirit we are invulnerable, in spite of what we are momentarily experiencing in our mind and body. If we gave up our identification with the body, and healed the conflict in our mind, we would be "safe and healed and whole" as *A Course in Miracles* states.

How can we give up fear if we are afraid to give up attack thoughts and judgment, which is made up of attack thoughts, as both generate fear? Another way to release fear is to forgive our grievances, because forgiveness heals fear.

We could also let go of the attachments we have, as all fear comes from fear of loss.

We could feel the emotion of fear until it evolves into a feeling of peace.

We could choose.

Some favorite lines about choice from *A Course in Miracles* are: "This need not be and I could have peace instead of this," and "There has to be a better way!" I use these as a mantra at times, focusing on the problems and removing the problem, layer by layer.

Another way to heal fear is to practice gratitude and appreciation; both put you in a flow which heals the fear.

Love heals fear. God as Love, created you as love. It is your essence. Revel in it. Spread it. Share it in every way you can think of.

Celebration also heals fear, though if there is more fear waiting in the deeper mind, it will come to the surface before you can fully enjoy the feeling of celebration. It is then important to take one more healing step to clear out all the fear that you have, impacted inside, on the way to celebration. Only when you know what the fear is about, can you transform it. Fear always has an object that will reveal itself if you dwell on it a moment.

Restore bonding; as you do so, the fear and split mind that began when you lost the bonding is healed. You can also give yourself fully to another as a way to help them and yourself. This level of commitment takes you to the next step beyond your fear. Heal your fear and you heal your pain. The resistance, that began with lost bonding and which generates the pain, is also dissolved as a result of willingness, which is one of the natural antidotes to fear and resistance. A step forward is a step forward in bonding.

In *A Course in Miracles* it also states that if you realized who walked with you, you could never be afraid.

In this lesson a number of ways to heal fear have been presented. Take time to practice all of them. Then as other problems surface you will be ready for them.

Lesson 79 – *Disconnection*

Pain, like illness, reflects a disconnection from oneself, and a disconnection from spirit. Dissolving the disconnection from yourself and spirit has the power to strengthen your health and feeling of wholeness. Disconnection from self causes a split mind with resulting conflicts. While disconnection from spirit is a disconnection from love, light and wholeness.

Disconnection for any reason is a mistake for which we will suffer. It sets up destructive patterns that continue on until resolved.

Ask yourself, if you were to know, what is the most important time you disconnected from yourself and now need to heal?

Who was there, if you were to know?

What was going on, that you disconnected from yourself?

When you disconnected at this time any adult in the scene was already disconnected from themselves, and any pain you suffered was pain that was already inside them. You can change this experience for everyone now, since minds are all connected. You will not allow attack from yourself or others if you are connected to yourself. First, reconnect with yourself. Then help everyone in that scene reconnect to themselves, so that attack of any kind falls away. Next, ask yourself intuitively what soul level gifts you brought in for everyone in that scene, to save them from themselves and to complete a soul level promise you made to do just that. Next, ask yourself what gifts Heaven had for those in that situation with you, to help save them from themselves. Open the door in your mind for your soul gifts and receive Heaven's gifts to share with whoever was in that situation with you.

Repeat this exercise once more with the second most important time that you disconnected from yourself.

When this is complete, ask yourself when it was that you disconnected from spirit in a significant way.

Ask yourself if it was in this life or another

If it was in this life, ask yourself, if you were to know, how old you were when you disconnected from spirit. Who was with you, if you were to know?

What was going on, if you were to know?

What led you to disconnect from spirit and wholeness?

If you will, reconnect to spirit and receive the gifts of spirit for yourself in that situation.

Now receive Heaven's gifts for the others in that situation.

How is that situation turning out now with that reconnection?

And how is the rest of your life turning out with that reconnection?

If it was a past life, ask yourself, what country you were living in, if you were to know

Ask yourself if you were a man or a woman

Ask yourself what was going on in that time and place, and what was the lesson you were looking to learn from it

What was it that occurred that disconnected you from the wholeness of your spirit, if you were to know?

What gift had you brought in at a soul level to contribute in that life?

What gift did Heaven want to give you for everyone in that life?

Receive Heaven's gifts, and open your own to share with everyone from the time you are a little child in that life. Consciously reconnect to Heaven and your spirit.

How does that life turn out now?

Bring the energy of that life into all of your lives since then and up to the present moment in this life.

How does that feel now?

Repeat this exercise with the second most important time in which you disconnected from spirit.

Lesson 80 – Faith

Faith is a powerful healing method which we can use to get ourselves back on track if we are suffering. Faith is using the natural power of the mind in a positive way. Suffering and pain speak of conflicts within us at subconscious and unconscious levels. Faith forges our mind back together by intent and will. It focuses on the outcome so completely that everything unfolds as we want it to.

Our faith is dragged down by belief systems to the contrary, and hidden selves that come from split minds. Yet choice is present and powerful, while beliefs which are made from old choices are static. This sometimes makes them harder to catch so that we can let go of them, but the power of faith uses the power of mind and the power of now, and it chooses again in a more positive vein.

When using faith to end pain you might begin by asking your higher mind to release all beliefs, hidden selves and ego attachments that have an investment in the status quo, and that make you have to suffer as a result. Ask that any lesson you need to learn to end your pain comes to you easily and gracefully.

Choose your outcome and know that being pain-free is in total alignment with God's Will for your happiness. Ask for nothing that is out of emotional integrity, such as asking for something that belongs to another. Ask for the truth. Do not ask for the end of suffering, which comes from your indulgence and hidden emotional attachment. Ask that you let these indulgences and attachments go, so you can not only be free of pain, but also experience love and happiness.

If you are undergoing emotional pain, choose the outcome in which the truth occurs and everyone wins.

Next, focus the power of your mind on a true and better outcome. Choose it. Commit to it. Want it until that is all that is in your mind. If another emotion or thought comes up that seems to go against the outcome, such as fear or some doubt, say to yourself: ***"This thought or feeling reflects a goal that is keeping me from my true outcome. I would rather have my true goal. Let it be as I have chosen."***

Next, concentrate on your desired outcome. See it as already accomplished. Feel it as if it is already accomplished, along with the sense of thanks that would go with your release from pain. If you think of it again, either repeat the process above, or simply know your outcome is on its way to you. Choose some believable time for yourself to have your goal accomplished, your desires fulfilled, and you to be free of pain.

Lesson 81 – Faith II

Faith is the power of your mind pointed in a positive direction. It is a choice that becomes an investment in the best possible outcome. The outcome of any situation shows where our faith has gone. Our mind has to be invested in something. A split mind results in a haphazard result. Jesus assured us that if we had faith the size of a mustard seed we could move mountains. Now mustard seeds are quite small, if you have ever seen one, certainly much smaller than a peppercorn. The point is that a little faith goes a long way. An unused mind is not just a waste; it becomes dangerous, for it becomes prey to every passing whim or vagary of the world and the collective ego. You can easily become part of the economic current or be tossed by the winds of war. This is not leadership or vision; it is being part of the herd. It is difficult being successful if you are a cultural conformist, because you are playing it safe like most people. Living in this way you become the natural prey of predators, especially if you lag behind the herd in any way.

Faith on the other hand sets your own course and, working in tandem with Heaven, you set the highest course. People are unfaithful or fail you when you are faithless in relationships, business or otherwise. This sets up power struggles and the failure of the ongoing business or relationship.

In this lesson, we will break down the steps in using the success principle of faith.

First, choose an area you would like to work on in regard to faith. It may be an area that is somewhat successful, an area of your life that is so-so, or an area of your life in which there is explicit fear or pain. The more fear or pain there is, the bigger the challenge and the bigger the reward. The key is to create not just a success in the area you have chosen, but a successful way of using this principle for ongoing success for the rest of your life. Let faith become a way of life. This is a powerful principle in a world where there is so much uncertainty. Once you have chosen the area you wish to concentrate on to use faith, reflect on your emotions, the circumstances working for and against you, and the current situation.

Imagine that negative emotions and circumstances, that seem to go against you, reflect your belief systems and parts of your mind that are going in a different direction to your ostensible goal. Ask Heaven to draw these emotions, belief systems and parts of your mind back to your center, which is a place of peace. Your center, with its peace and grace, melts away anything that is not peaceful. It is this peace that gives rise to the faith that brings success in every circumstance. A peaceful mind generates confidence, and confidence generates success.

If any untoward emotions, circumstances or thoughts seem to pop up again, ask Heaven that they be returned to the center of your mind, where they will melt back into pure potential to be used in a positive way.

Your next step is to choose the highest possible outcome, in alignment with success and truth. Ask Heaven's help in inspiring you with the highest outcome. Now put your mind to have this outcome occur. Again, any negative thoughts, emotions or circumstances reflect hidden belief systems and parts of your mind. They may even be coming through the collective but it can still be healed personally. The peace at the center of your mind becomes ever more pure with each *centering* you ask for.

Spend five minutes to begin with, **knowing** that the outcome you wish for is yours. You deserve it. It is God's Will for you, so know it *now* as what will soon occur. It is not so important that each little thing that you choose is the way you want it to be. What is important is the success of you using the principle of faith, until it becomes a way of life for you and so becomes the heart of your success.

Let the positive outcome be a touchstone that your mind goes back to again and again. Bring back to your center any thoughts that are other than the thought of success.

Finally, allow yourself gratitude for the outcome that is about to occur. It is this sense of thanksgiving that not only creates flow, it tells your mind that the outcome has already been accomplished as you have imagined it.

The ego attempts to sabotage anything that is a natural principle of success such as faith - a God-given gift that is a function of the mind. For instance, the ego substitutes naiveté for faith as a way to wreak havoc and delay us. Naiveté is a form of denial. It blithely ignores the signs and signals that something is amiss. There is hell to pay as a result, and it shows itself as business defeat, heartbreak or bankruptcy depending on the arena. This, of course, is the opposite of what faith brings about. You can provide an antidote to naiveté through awareness, and by asking that anything you may be blind to, be shown to you by your own higher mind or Heaven.

So, choose your area.

Choose your outcome.

Bring to your center anything that is not success.

Know your result.

Be thankful for your result.

Ask that anything hidden that could stop or delay you be brought to your awareness and your center.

Enjoy the result.

Lesson 82 – Your Angel

My favorite picture of an angel is one that comes to me from my childhood. Above the blackboard behind the nun's desk, there was a long picture of an angel, arms spread in protection as a couple of children crossed a rickety bridge over a stream with a few planks missing. It seemed night was coming on or there was the lowering sky of an incoming storm. Yet with the angel, there was a sense of safety. "No problem," the picture seemed to say. God's security agency is on the job. Even today, I can recall that picture with a fondness.

Heaven knows I had some close calls: in the water, in planes, at sports, freefalling down a stairwell. Numerous times I could have been killed or paralyzed. I believe my angel worked overtime for any number of years.

Most of us go blithely through our lives. Especially when we reach the stage of independence, we seem to imagine that we are doing everything by ourselves. Yet, if we bypassed this stage, we would develop interdependence with others and with Heaven. Angels can then come back into vogue as messengers, guides and celestial security agents. It is this last role that I would especially like to address.

Your angel would, by definition of what an angel is, love you. Your angel would be your protector. Your angel, unless overridden by soul pattern or hidden choice, seeks to save you from yourself and from mistakes that lead you towards death and away from God. It would be in your best interest to be in alignment with your angel. Your happiness depends on it. When you get yourself caught in a painful trap, your angel works to get your attention to show you the way out.

In my fanciful mind, every time an angel succeeds in guiding us to make the right choice, they get a feather for their wings. Unfortunately, most of our angels look like supermarket chickens.

This is a good time to spend getting to know your angel. Build a relationship. Get to know this light being. Listen to their wise counsel. Ask them to make it clear to you what went on in your mind that led to the pain. Ask the best way out. Ask that your inner conflict and fear be removed. Help your angel to move you out of the category of hard cases. You have a friend in a high place and they are your bridge from Heaven to Earth. Enjoy your 'Fire Lord,' your luminous friend. Let them help you to make your life easier.

Lesson 83 – Being the Cause

We understand that we are the cause of our dreams, in spite of the fact that they seemingly come to us without any will of our own. We are the dreamer of the dreams, not only in our night-time, but also in our daytime. This is not a path for everyone, but those who tread the path of accountability become more responsible for their lives. It gives us back our power and we become the cause of the lives we live, rather than the effect of the world. Taking responsibility allows us to see the direct correlation between our world and what is happening in our mind. As we change our mind, we can change our world.

In the 1970's I learned as many dream therapies as I could and reveled in using them to free clients of deep patterns but by the 1980's I had learned that our lives were also a dream. As such, they readily lent themselves to all of the dream therapy models. After that discovery, I used these models as readily for what was occurring in our lives in the daytime as I did for the stories we dreamed at night. Simply owning that you are the cause, rather than that you are the victim of the world you experience, begins to transform any negative event.

Spend time today taking responsibility for your life. You do not have to believe this. You do not even have to accept it. Yet consider this principle. Examine this principle. Pretend this principle is true. Pretend that the most fundamental principle of dream therapy, that dreams are wish fulfillment, is true and that your life is your 'waking dream.' You may not believe it. You may strongly believe it is not true. Yet this principle can still benefit you.

Pretend that you wished to have the pain you have.

How come?

Why would you possibly want the pain?

We know you don't want it, but somehow pretend that you do. How could that be?

Hang out with this idea all day long. Dwell on it. How could this be?

Take some real time to examine your life in terms of this principle.

Lesson 84 – The Wrong Perception of Pain

I was doing my morning lessons in *A Course in Miracles* and I came to Lesson 190:

"I choose the joy of God instead of pain."
Here is the first paragraph:

"Pain is a wrong perspective. When it is experienced in any form, it is a proof of self-deception. It is not a fact at all. There is no form it takes that will not disappear if seen aright. For pain proclaims God cruel. How could it be real in any form? It witnesses to God the Father's hatred of His Son, the sinfulness He sees in him and His insane desire for revenge and death."

Of course, God is Love and only what is loving proceeds from Him. He is not insane and does not thirst for revenge and death.

"Pain is a wrong perspective." I have found this to be true both psychologically and spiritually. It is a wrong perception psychologically because guilt, fear, revenge, loss and control, which are a few of the key dynamics of any type of pain, are psychological mistakes. Being mistakes, they can be corrected and transformed by the forgiveness, bonding, and love that reflect truth.

Spiritually, pain is also a mistake and not a fact. Pain denies we are spirit, declaring we are bodies. Pain is meant to prove God is the ultimate 'Bad Guy' and that He is out for our blood because of His hatred and judgment of us. Neither these feelings nor revenge can be true of Love, Light or Spirit. Unless, of course, there is a theology so skewed that it declares our pain is good and our death is God's Will. Pain and death are ultimate weapons of the ego, declaring God is bad and that **we** should be God, being ultimately more powerful than God since we can die and God cannot stop it. The ego, out of its projection of guilt, is always out to frame God and blame Him for the terrible self-punishment that our pain is. One can live a happy, fulfilled life, living by any religion, especially if love, forgiveness and letting go of judgments are emphasized. People have reached sanctity and enlightenment from almost every spiritual path there is.

But at times, certain religious paths become too restrictive and repressive, emphasizing psychological mistakes as the way forward. When people can no longer stand to be bound by such strictures, they leave and look for another path.

"To go beyond the ego and its body identification is to go beyond pain and know the joy of God. We have all deceived ourselves into thinking we are a body because we have identified with our ego"

Now let us switch allegiance. Now let us give up this "dream of fierce retaliation for a crime that could not be committed."

If we are spirit, we cannot be guilty because only Oneness is the reality. We can only dream we acted badly and deserve to suffer.

Even psychologically, dreams of guilt are dreams of specialness. We make it all about us but not in a good way. We have dreamed that we are bad, even evil, but dreams do not leave the mind. It is true that one body can inflict damage on another body, but it is like one car crashing into another. The car that crashed into another is not guilty. Displacing mind problems onto the body will cause psychological and physical pain, but when the conflict of the mind is healed, no pain remains.

To end pain by healing the conflict of the mind is to create peace and health. Yet, sooner or later, another conflict will come up, given the tens of thousands of self-concepts we have, each one vying for its own personal brand of happiness. Sooner or later, to escape the pain, we must escape the dream. To wake up to God's Love, and our own, is waking up to the creation and extension of God's Love. Awakening, not death, is the way out of pain. Whether it be the small awakening that leads out of a particular pain or the big Awakening out of the dream, it is one that helps us remember that both we and God are innocent, and we no longer need blame God for our perceived sins.

When our guilt is gone there is nothing to project on others or on God. When we blame ourselves for something, then we will have judgments and grievances toward others to hide our guilt. You cannot have a judgment or grievance against someone unless there is a self-concept within you that is similar to what you judge in them. Otherwise, there is only compassion and a desire to help. Those we have projected on are helpful to us because they show us buried subconscious and unconscious guilt, as evidenced by our self-concepts.

Make a list of those you are close to who have wounded you or who have a problem, a character defect, or some kind of negativity. Next make a list of the qualities in them you have judgment on.

Then go through a number of exercises:

Experience the quality as yours. Accept it. Forgive it. Bless it. Let it go. Imagine it melting back into you as pure light.

Do not go onto the next step until you complete each step.

This first step may be difficult if you have compensated for a certain behavior, as you will have a role to hide this belief about yourself, but the very resistance lets you know there is something to hide. Winning back and healing something you have compensated for will create flow where you were stuck and unable to receive. For instance, once you experience some behavior as yours, only then go to accept it.

So the exercise should look something like this:

Judged Person _____

Judged Behaviors
1. _____ 2. _____ 3. _____

A. Experience it.

B. Accept it.

C. Forgive it.

D. Bless it.

E. Integrate it.

Remember you have suppressed or repressed these negative qualities to hide your guilt. These beliefs about yourself may be well defended by dissociation or compensation that you are now paying for with pain. Burn through the dissociation by aggressively feeling the resistance, numb or dead feeling.

The extent of the emotion defended against will be shown by the amount of resistance or dissociation. Sometimes you will go through a big process with many emotions before you come to peace and a new level of openhearted love. But such births are priceless in getting your heart back and opening your ability to receive. Healing these self-concepts that you never stopped punishing yourself for allows a big step forward.

Lesson 85 – Pain is Illusion

Fundamentally, we can have either illusions or truth but we cannot have both. When we lose bonding and experience separation instead of truth, we build our ego. Pain is a by-product of the separation of the ego. When we lose the love, success and ease that comes with bonding, we want it back. Only now, we have a split mind which generates fear. One part wants love, success and ease while the other wants independence, control and separation. This results in conflict and resistance, both of which give rise to pain.

When we lose bonding, we have illusion instead of joining. We do not see issues in their proper light because we are no longer looking at them through love and innocence. We are looking at them through judgment and fear and, as a result, we see illusion and separation, which if not immediately synonymous with pain soon become so.

One way to heal the separation using the mind is to ask yourself how many situations would need to be rebonded for you to have greater truth and be pain free.

If you were to know, it's probably

If you were to know when the latest one occurred, it's probably when you were at the age of

If you were to know who was involved, it was probably

If you were to know what occurred, it was probably

Now go to the light, deep within you, and join light to light with whoever is a part of that situation. Connect up everyone's light. How is the situation now?

Once again, join with everyone, light to light, and see how things seem as a result.

Do this until either everyone is in profound peace or the whole situation has turned to light.

Next, ask yourself when the previous situation of lost bonding and pain occurred.

It was probably at the age of

And if you were to know who was involved, it was probably

And if you were to know what occurred, it was probably

Once again, from your light connect everyone with light. Do this until it is complete.

Now go further back to the next problem and repeat the exercise.

This restores the bonding that frees you of pain. You may go back to situations in early childhood, at birth, in the womb, an ancestral situation, another lifetime, or even a story from the collective unconscious, when what is occurring does not directly involve you. No matter what the story, use your light and connect.

Spiritually, you can let God remove all of the blocks or beliefs between you and your experience of yourself as spirit. When this occurs, you will know yourself as love and feel the Love of God, and the illusion of pain dissolves.

Lesson 86 – Pain as the Denial of God

If God is Love and only that which is peaceful can come from God then pain is the opposite of God. It is a denial of love. As *A Course in Miracles* states:

> "It [pain] demonstrates God is denied, confused with fear, perceived as mad, and seen as a traitor to Himself. If God is real, there is no pain. If pain is real, there is no God. For vengeance is not part of love. And fear, denying love and using pain to prove that God is dead, has shown that death is victor over life. The body is the Son of God, corruptible in death, as mortal as the Father he has slain."

Of course, many of us believe in God but are suffering. Yet, is our God one of belief or experience? Have we felt Divine Love, or just taken it as part of our belief system? God is no belief and will not be limited by belief. However, if we look at what we think about God being in charge of our death then, in our belief, we think God is homicidal, wanting the suffering and death of His son. How could this be? Any loving father would want the best for their child. How much more so God! God is not schizophrenic that He would be Love and yet want someone's suffering and death, much less His Son's. We are schizophrenic and project it on God. He could not want suffering, sacrifice and martyrdom and be sane. He is the Supreme Force of Love and Purity. Only innocence could proceed from Him. As the Course remonstrates with us, it is time to give up our attack and investment in beliefs that we are full of "savage crimes or secret sins with weighty consequence."

It is through attack that the ego keeps itself alive. If we give up attack thoughts and value harmlessness, the ego becomes legless. Only innocence could proceed from the Innocence Itself that God is. The rest is a mad investment in an insane illusion, to which pain is witness. Once we have stopped long enough to consider our beliefs, and how they have set up a consensual reality that makes pain normal and suffering the status quo, we realize we can choose what we want our reality to be. Our separation is so profound that, at this point, we have literally constituted a world of illusion from separation. It is a world of suffering brought about from judgment and self-judgment. Yet, once we stop denying God, then our illusions and their repercussions of pain become laughable.

Today, ask for an experience of Divine Presence. Offer up your denial and invite in the Love of God that brings the peace that surpasses understanding. Open yourself to be profoundly touched and illumined. Let yourself be cradled in the Mind of God. Put your cares and worries in the Hands of God. Let yourself rest in expectancy. There is nothing to do today but invite in the Source of All That Is. Claim what is your heritage and your destiny. God will come to you through the power of His Love. There is nothing to do but accept.

Lesson 87 – Your Thoughts Alone

This lesson is once again about the power of your mind. Your thoughts are not insignificant and no thought is neutral. They either head toward suffering and death, or toward joy and life. Thoughts are things. They are investments in the world you look upon. They will either reflect a fearful self-image, or reflect the peace and love that is your essence.

To recognize the power of your mind is to take responsibility for it. The power of the mind denies guilt, as untrue and simply another form of attack on ourselves and as a way to fight God. To think you are responsible and to deny guilt is to give you back your power, and to give your mind to Heaven for guidance. It helps you awaken from the dream of separation and the nightmare of a world of pain. Fully embraced, accountability would bring enlightenment. If there was no blame and no guilt, we would realize our original state of mind, which is spirit. In our freedom, we would bless the world by carrying the awareness of our Self, God and Heaven wherever we go. The world around us would reflect the Heaven within us. A Course in Miracles expresses the power of our mind, thus:

> "It is your thoughts alone that cause you pain. Nothing external to your mind can hurt or injure you in any way. There is no cause beyond yourself that can reach down and bring oppression. No one but yourself affects you. There is nothing in the world that has the power to make you ill or sad, weak or frail. But it is you who have the power to dominate all things you see by merely recognizing what you are."

I had discovered this concept of accountability, and how it is our own mind that causes what occurs, in 1974 when I first began studying hypnosis. Later, in 1975, I developed the Intuitive Method as a way to get into the deeper mind for what was hidden there. When I first heard the term accountability, in a workshop in 1977, it helped me understand my near death experience and a number of close calls I had had with death.

I began to realize that guilt was a fallacy used to support the ego, but that responsibility on the other hand was empowering. It allowed us dominion over our world and it returned to us the responsibility for what was in our mind, because the world reflected what was there.

The Course goes on to say:

"The world you see does nothing. It has no effects at all. It merely represents your thoughts. And it will change entirely as you elect to change your mind, and choose the joy of God as what you really want."

There are thoughts that come from our wishes and they are conscious. There are thoughts in our subconscious that include what was really going on in our victim situations, which we don't find acceptable and hide. There are judgments we have made on ourselves that we buried, as well as old choices that have become beliefs, and therefore beliefs about ourselves. There are unconscious or soul patterns that also form our belief systems. There are ancestral belief systems that are also key for us. Beyond this, our thoughts are not our thoughts but come into our mind from the collective unconscious of humanity or the collective ego. Thoughts can also come from the demonic or dark unconscious of the astral. Even though all these thoughts are not our own as such, we can take responsibility and make choices around them, such as letting go or choosing the thoughts of our higher mind instead. We need not let ourselves be directed by dark thoughts of attack.

Today ask to be shown where your thinking is off. Ask to be shown vividly the thoughts that have led to your current pain. Take some time to meditate on this and let this question be on your mind all day. Ask to be shown in such a way that you can't miss it. Ask this with all your heart. It's your mind. Claim what you want from it.

When the answer does come to you about what led to the pain, turn it over to your higher mind and the Holy Spirit to undo what got you into trouble. Spend time listening for the way out. Heaven always has a way out and will respond to your calls for help and healing.

Lesson 88 – Shamanic Tests

We all go through tests in life. These challenges are not just tests of memory or the intellect. They are tests of the mind and heart. Some are small tests, such as, will we be kind or cruel in our response to someone, or will we take a step closer to someone or a step into further separation. Most of these tests are small without major or immediate results or repercussions.

On the other hand, there are some tests that have been set up by the soul, even before we came into this life. If we succeed in them, it is as if we are initiated into a new level of power, love or success. Our mind and heart expand. Our creativity and psychic power grow. To fail a soul level test whether self-initiated, given by a teacher or brought on by a sudden onslaught of life at its worst or most demanding, can generate some of the worst pain in our lives.

Tests like these were frequently given by shamans to their apprentices. This could show up as a life or death situation, such as drinking a certain liquid that could kill you, drive you insane or have you step beyond the boundaries of the natural world. Other initiations could come upon a person seemingly unbidden, such as an illness or accident. In some of the illnesses, a person might see themselves, or a certain part of the body such as the eyes, devoured by demons. If the person survived the illness they would find they had a facility in healing or, as in the case of the demon who devoured their eyes, a gift in healing eye maladies. Shamanic power could sometimes be opened up when a person, in the face of threat or need, would rise up and open some long lost ability that would save the day.

Typically, the shaman was asked to venture everything and, heroically, put it all on the line. They would expand to greater consciousness and use shamanic gifts which are beyond the ken of everyday life.

In our lives, we have from time to time set up shamanic tests. If we pass them, we achieve a new level of confidence, with the power to have a new stage of success because of the expansion of our heart and mind. If we flunk these tests, we feel barely alive or that our heart has been ripped from our chest. Tests we flunked are ongoing. They remain inside us until we pass the test, but usually they are buried under major dissociation so we can survive while feeling that much pain. When we flunk a shamanic test, we seem diminished from our previous greatness, and walk with lesser stature. But once we realize that the test is ongoing, we can retake and pass it.

What it takes to pass a shamanic test is:

1. Giving ourselves wholeheartedly; putting it all on the line.
2. Forgiveness.
3. Asking Heaven's help.

Giving It All

If you give it all, and then give some more of what you didn't know you had, your mind expands and what you thought was possible grows. Vision opens and a way is made clear. Powers long hidden open in a natural way for the situation at hand.

Forgiveness

There is a line from *A Course in Miracles* which states: "I will forgive, and this will disappear." First, begin by forgiving yourself and then the situation. Then forgive every person in the situation, and what is going wrong. Forgive everyone and everything past and present. Forgive your split mind that perceives the situation, and forgive the conflict. You can forgive away a shamanic test layer by layer but, if any hidden unforgiveness remains, so will the suffering or threat. Ask your higher mind to find and forgive what is necessary for you to pass the test.

Asking Heaven's Help

Asking for a miracle, considered by some to be cheating in the best possible way, is the easy way to pass a shamanic test. It puts everything back in perspective, helping us remember we are God's precious child and deserve all good things easily. Ask with all your heart for a miracle, as God hears your heart not your words.

A shamanic test, when passed, integrates major splits in the unconscious mind. There can be ongoing shamanic tests, such as when one's parents are at war. At one level, the emotional pressure can turn your life to rubble, or the pressure can make you into a diamond. If you pass a shamanic test in this regard, you become a diamond that helps others become diamonds.

Examine your life now for times you felt you had your heart ripped out, and you barely escaped with your life. They are the most painful events of your life.

List these events for yourself.

1. ....
2. ....
3. ....

Then ask yourself, how much of each test you passed in terms of percentage. The rest is what you have yet to learn.

Now, pick a method from the three mentioned and practice it until you are at peace and feel the creative might or shamanic gift inside you that comes of passing such a test.

Remember, if you still feel pain or judgment on anything, there will be some vestiges left to complete. These shamanic tests were set up by you – your very soul. You must have confidence at some deep level that you can pass the test and that there is a way. Don't give up. There is a better way and you can find it.

In terms of healing pain in your life, know that there is a way out. Ask before you sleep, and when you wake up, that the root events be shown to you. Healing root events can give you a "leg up" when it comes to passing a shamanic test. Give to everyone and everything as much as you can. Forgive every upset in the past to free the present. Ask for the miracle to pass the test and ask for the grace to do it easily.

Lesson 89 – Harmlessness

"As you perceive the harmlessness in them [things in the world], they will accept your holy will as theirs. And what was seen as fearful now becomes a source of innocence and holiness."

Harmlessness is a mastery level quality that goes hand in hand with compassion. It is the end of attack which is the very foundation of the ego so that, as a result, there is movement beyond conflict and into joy. This moves us into the profound peace that is beyond dualism and into the unity of the mind.

For us to perceive harmlessness in another, there must be harmlessness in ourselves because the law of perception is such that we look in before we look out. If we are harmless, we will see harmlessness in others and, if we do, they will join us in harmlessness because our will is more whole and therefore holy and irresistible. The beauty of innocence is enchanting because the world has become safe.

Forgiveness renders us harmless and therefore helpful in a situation where judgment could have turned attack into grievance. We are neither predator nor prey, no longer attracted to death but generating life. The dominion that comes of our holy will, our spirit, leads those around us back to their own spirit so that they might know their own harmlessness and holiness.

Blessings and helpfulness proceed from harmlessness contributing to peace in the world. It is a simple way of being that does so much good. To be harmless we must be peaceful. To be peaceful we must forgive all that angers, irritates or upsets us. Otherwise, we add fuel to the fire. Harmlessness welcomes. It takes responsibility. The buck stops here and anger and pain are transformed, rather than increased and passed on.

Let yourself possess the utter attractiveness of innocence. Be masterful with those around you. Let blessings and beauty abound. Your harmlessness expunges your guilt; it makes you safe and extends your safety to those around you.

Your harmlessness, which is what would make you a bridge between Heaven and Earth, goes beyond your ego.

To free your mind of harm is to be pain free and brings that harmlessness to everyone around you.

Today practice harmlessness. Let go of every irritation, upset and anger. Know your forgiveness will free you of every temptation to react and so increase your own pain. Today police your mind for any anger or irritation, past and present. Extend yourself in forgiveness rather than withdraw in judgment. Let the buck stop with you. Burn through any negative emotion till you are at peace and it is released from the world. You choose between freedom or being in a prison of pain. Let the past go and commit to harmlessness that you might be set free.

Lesson 90 – The Lesson of Pain

Pain is an indicator that we have not learned a certain lesson. Both an understanding and a place where we have not forgiven, have evaded us. If the understanding comes to us, then forgiveness is assured because with the fullness of understanding, bonding is restored and grievances are released. When forgiveness is employed, bonding is restored and the lesson is learned.

If we are suffering, we are caught in an illusion that causes us pain. We can ask for the understanding that will free us. We have the right to claim the truth for ourselves. Heaven wants us to have the truth. The only thing in the way is our ego, also an illusion of separation that we have invested in and thus given meaning and value. It shrieks in fear that we will die, but it is our ego that will die, bit by bit, as truth and understanding come. Forgiveness helps us see that what was wounded was the ego, an idea of ourselves that is not worth defending. Forgiveness helps us realize that there was no insult, only someone that needed our help and if we don't extend the help, we will suffer inside as they have.

Now let us invoke the power of forgiveness. *A Course in Miracles* calls forgiveness 'love on the earthly plane.' Negativity, pain and perception are transformed through forgiveness.

> "How can you tell when you are seeing wrong, or someone else is failing to perceive the lesson he should learn? Does pain seem real in the perception? If it does, be sure the lesson is not learned. And there remains an unforgiveness hiding in the mind that sees the pain through eyes the mind directs."

It goes on to say that lessons are God's way of removing all that would hurt us, leaving not one unforgiving thought unhealed, nor nails or thorns left over to hurt us. God would have all unshed tears released and wiped away, and have laughter replace each of these that we be free once more.

Today, spend significant time in the morning and evening forgiving any anger, upset, grievance or perceived failures on another's part. Let mercy and truth be yours. Forgive the pain. Forgive those trying to help. Forgive your enemies or those you projected on as the perpetrator of this pain. When this is complete, go to your past. What you see others doing or failing to do is what you are doing or failing to do. When you get through your denial you will see it and, if you continue to see, you will begin to break your contract with the ego that contains your death in the small print.

Forgive all the pain of the past. Forgive yourself as the one who set up the lesson but has not learned it. Forgive the people and situations of past upset and pain. Let understanding and peace be yours today.

Every hour spend some time on what remains of the pain and the present situation. Especially examine the period of six months to two years before any chronic pain began, to find grievances with people and events in the root situation which led to this chronic pain. Let this be a day of forgiveness and freedom for you and for those you forgive, who no longer have to bear the burden of your projection. Even if a hundred people have the same projection on a person, your forgiveness might be strong enough to transform the perception, not just for you and the one you were angry with, but for everyone. Use the Course's forgiveness exercise today:

"I will forgive, and this will disappear."

Your present situation may be chronic and impacted but each forgiveness moves you closer and closer to being pain free, having learned the lesson.

Lesson 91 – Freeing the Future

To free the future is to transcend every conflict of the mind. When there is no past conflict, there is no pain. Nothing is dragged from the past to the present or future as punishment for sins believed in. Grief and misery, as well as pain and loss, fall away when the past is healed. There is no longer an investment in separation, so you remove yourself from the rack of time by freeing your future. The illusions of the past are no longer and, as a result, fear of the future falls away. When fear stops, separation ends and the fallacy of guilt gives way to innocence and a unity that is love and abundance.

King guilt and queen sorrow are removed from their usurped thrones, and the rightful heirs of peace and beauty are returned to their thrones. All this occurs when the future is freed from the slavery of the past. Psychology fades away, as do excuses. All that is left is a transcendent now, a doorway to the light, a time saver and a life saver.

How all this is accomplished is by simply placing your future in the Hands of God. How this is handled is simply to place the past in the Hands of God. How could there be worry or fear when what is coming is handled by your Beloved, who loves you more than you could ever imagine love to be? Placing your past and future in the Hands of God wrecks the ego's need for the illusion of continuity, which it uses to shuttle pain from one moment to the next.

The ego fuses time together for the purpose of pain, and so to motivate your death. Without the ego's sleight of hand in regard to time, we would have each moment standing clear and singing an eternal now and an eternal *new* that would lead you to experience a beginner's mind with sweet wonder. You would no longer need the control of the ego; you would always be falling in love and as you fall in love, your heart and mind would be open to the inexorable pull of Heaven. In no one moment can you suffer pain. In no one moment can you die. In no one moment can you experience loss, but the ego has condemned you to "doing time" on death row. Fusing time means the inexorable suffering goes on without relief. Putting the past and future in God's Hands is to return time to God to unfold it gently and easily for you as you return to Oneness and its exquisite joy.

To give God your future is to give Him your past and the present as well. You begin letting go of your burdens one by one. You see the way to perfect peace, unfolding before you step by step. To give God your past and future is to allow help, and the grace you need, to come to you. To give God your future is to take the crown off your ego, and its voracious need for significance, and to give it back to God who has already bestowed inestimable value on you.

This lesson from *A Course in Miracles* about placing the future in God's Hands, has always been one of my favorites. It gives me peace because I know I don't have to worry about the outcome. It is not just handled, it is handled by the Hand of God. I recognize I have no need for the stress of attempting to control every little thing. I can relax and enjoy myself even when big issues are at hand.

The more you practice this lesson of freeing the future, the more the ego is dissembled and God takes over. The Great Friend has come to help and you can surrender yourself and your future into those loving Hands.

Free your future and you free yourself of pain, because there is nothing to fear and no reason to attack yourself for a past that never was; it was only imagined. Place your future in the Hands of God and let yourself be loved.

Lesson 92 – Over the Years

Over the years, in my own personal and professional life, I learned that when I was upset I was ultimately upset with myself. Peace became more and more valuable to me. I learned that if I forgave everyone, myself included, along with the situation and even *things* that upset me, I would be returned, layer by layer, to ever deeper peace. A *Course in Miracles* states it most succinctly for me:

> "Do not forget today that there can be no form of suffering that fails to hide an unforgiving thought. Nor can there be a form of pain forgiveness cannot heal."

Today, go through your life, year by year and person by person. Start from the present and go backwards or start from your conception and come forward. Forgive everyone and everything. You'll find that you have judgments even on those you were closest to. Forgive them all. Take it year by year. Go at your own pace. It may take a few hours or it may take a month. Forgive problems and situations. Forgive the people in them. Forgive yourself. Forgive life. Forgive God.

Lesson 93 – The Self-Deception of Fear

I have already written of how fear began when bonding was lost. And I have further written about how bonding was not so much lost, as broken by us to gain freedom. But breaking bonding with its incumbent pain is like breaking out of prison on the day your sentence was to be commuted. Now, you are always on the run and constantly looking over your shoulder. All this occurred because, on the day you were to be freed, you had another plan. Listening to the ego's advice you mistook independence for freedom. Now, there is all hell to pay, and the ego demands its pound of pain in order to keep the self-deception going. No one traumatized you. You chose it in order to separate, constructing personalities which were built around the victim, sacrificer and rebel. This is not who you are. You have covered over your relatedness with pain and self-concepts. You have denied your *being* so you know yourself not so much as a *human being* but as a *human doing*.

You weren't the victim and you are not even the sacrificer and the rebel. These are personalities you have put on to hide your Self. You are God's Child. You know this more and more as you give up your traumas, with their hidden tantrums and rebellion. You are God's Child and He would not wish on you what you have wished on yourself. And if you believe, in the deepest recesses of your mind, that someone else wounded you, you believe God did the same thing. If you believe that a parent abandoned you, did not want you or broke your heart, you believe that God must have done the same thing to you. How could that be? You have deceived yourself and framed God and others for your abandonment, for you not wanting them, and for you breaking your own heart by rejecting them.

You believe you are a self that could never be. And so you look upon a world that could not be. Nothing in the world could be true because it only reflects your own self-deceiving concepts. Do not believe these illusions. They bring a scarcity of love and success to your world. Don't spend your life witnessing a world that is not true, nor telling a life story that is a tragic fantasy. God could not wish this on you and remain Love.

Fear is not real. We are the Child of God Himself. Fear is self-deception and you need not invest in foolish fear any longer. Pain, and the fear that drives it, could not be God's Will for you. Want what God wants for you. Know yourself as God knows you. Accept His miracles. Pardon others and you will be pardoned yourself. Give up independence for the partnership you are offered. These offers will continue until you experience unity both within and without. These offers will continue until you embrace union once more and can commune with God and All That Is.

This will continue until, once again, you realize your Oneness. Why not now?

Why wait for Heaven when the rest is self-deception and God Himself is reaching down to you, wanting you to have a Heaven on Earth Story?

Lesson 94 – Pain is Misperception

All healing takes place on the level of perception. It comes from the mind and is then reflected in every other area of our lives. If it does not take place on this level, then what occurs is merely the replacement of one symptom of pain with another. When we are in pain, misperception is occurring in regard to someone around us, in regard to ourself and in regard to God. To clear any one of these levels totally is to be free of pain

When we blame another for our present state, it is in an effort to avoid responsibility for what is occurring. We have misperceived some situation and their call for help. As a result, we did not learn the lesson that would have empowered us. We did not open the soul level gift we brought into this life especially for the situation, and instead chose self-concepts that have led to pain. Now we are invested in a story that did not take place and a self that is not us. The original situation breeds patterns of misperception about us and others, leading to many levels of pain.

We have also misperceived God. In the deep unconscious, we blame God for our situation, depicting Him as cruel and demanding our punishment. Our pain states that He is not a loving Father at all, but One Who hates us. We hide these notions from ourselves as they could not bear the scrutiny of reason.

What heals misperception is the desire to be no longer imprisoned by illusion. Any of the following healing principles, to name a few, give us right perception:

1. Forgive the significant other you blame for this. Forgive yourself. Forgive life. Forgive God.
2. Let go of your hidden indulgence, both physical and emotional. This painful situation hides an emotional indulgence.
3. Embrace your gift for the current situation, and another soul gift for the significant past situation that led to this. Share this gift with those around you.
4. Accept God's gifts. His Love and His miracles are here to free you, His beloved child.
5. Your trust would unravel the situation that has become tangled to generate this painful conflict.

6. Give up judgment and, instead, increasingly bless.
7. Commit to the next step with all your heart. The next step is *always* better than this one, in spite of what your ego tells you.
8. Ask that your perception, both now and in the past, be replaced with peace.

Lesson 95 – The Idol of Cruelty

Idols are hidden goals that we have made into gods. Through these false gods, we seek our happiness and our salvation. More powerful, insidious and hidden than an addiction, an idol has the ability to negate all the positive aspects of manifesting, prayer, claiming, wanting something with all our heart and other aspects of mind power that can open us to peace and healing. An idol is a trump card the ego uses to deny the power of the mind for healing. Idols are hidden deep in the personal unconscious and not readily accessible. Many times, they are compensated for, such as when someone who is quite repressed has an idol of sex, or when a person in scarcity represses an idol of money.

Over the years, I have gotten a little better at finding them but mostly I use my process healing cards to find when they have been having an effect on the situation. Over the years, I have developed healing card decks as a way of exploring subconscious and unconscious dynamics, and the healing, gift and grace available to us in any situation.

There is a principle in *A Course in Miracles* that, when I read it, struck me as so psychologically true as to be worth immediate learning: anything we wish on another we become vulnerable to. Even though dark wishes do not leave our mind, and illusions have no real effect except in the world of illusions, yet what we wish on others we become open to ourselves. So if we have cruel wishes or attack thoughts on others, we believe that we are open to cruelty and attack ourselves. Having Idols of Cruelty thus makes us heir to cruel things happening to us, and this includes pain. We do not escape what we wish on others for good or ill. Having Idols of Cruelty means we are constantly wishing others and ourselves to suffer, in order to make offerings to these gods of darkness.

If you will, ask yourself how many Idols of Cruelty you have within you.

It is probably

Imagine you are entering the temple of your mind and walking to the very center, where your altar is. This is where you make offerings to Heaven, life and others. There you will find your Idols of Cruelty. With Heaven's help, knock them off your altar. They will be immediately replaced with the lilies of forgiveness. Also, a light will shine down on the middle of your altar and another gift will appear there. Enjoy these gifts and let them become part of your life. If you do not understand what a certain gift means, simply ask Heaven its meaning.

Lesson 96 – Ask Today What God Wills for You

In the Bible, it suggests that we pray, and pray unceasingly. Let today be such a day.

First of all, no friend, worthy of the name, would want their friend to be in pain. If that is true, then how could the great Friend want anything less for you. So today, as you ask to be free of suffering, recognize that you ask for what God Wills for you. It is only a matter of getting your will in alignment with God's. Your true will, beyond your ego, wants no pain because this will came from God's Will. Your ego's will, which obviously you have identified with, doesn't really care if you suffer or not. As a matter of fact, suffering is what the ego uses for getting attention, dark glamour and significance, even though it is to our own detriment. Today identify with your true Self. Crack open your mind and heart, and receive the love from your Friend. Love and comfort are always given by the Friend. Now be open to the bounty and grace that your Friend has for you, and pray unceasingly that you may come into alignment with God's Will for you.

Lesson 97 – Pain as Obsession

When we are in pain, we obsess about it. It captures our attention so vividly that, at times, it has the power to block out most other experiences. I have found that anything we obsess about is a trap. Even if we are obsessing about a good thing, it takes us out of the flow and we do not move forward. Anything that delays us is a trap. Even if we are thinking of our beloved to the point of obsession, we are using them to hold ourselves back.

It is obvious that pain is an obsession, and it is obvious that it is a trap. I have found that all of the things that generate obsession, such as addiction, humiliation, taboos, and social caste, are there to keep us from hearing the guidance within. This is an inspiration given to us for a leadership project that has to do with a function our soul has set up for our benefit, and the world's benefit.

Our pain is a way of bowing and scraping as an excuse. It is the arrogance of false humility. It is the running away from our purpose. But, if we are called to do a certain project, then we have the strength for it and the help of grace as well. If we are called to do it, and we open ourselves to the inspiration and guidance, then we can accomplish it, no matter how great it is. Our minds and our hearts are perfectly suited to what we have been assigned. It is in our best interest to accept our function, because the pain is a defense, an attempt to overwhelm and distract us from what we are called for. Accepting our vocation has the ability either to dissolve the pain altogether, or have it lessen step by step, as we embrace what we have been called to do. We have the gifts that can free the world and, if there is anything else that is necessary, Heaven will give it to us to give as it is needed.

Today, ask what it is that you are called to do. Let your willingness be your prayer. Step away from your pain today as you embrace the assignments your soul has for you.

Lesson 98 – Pain and God

God lives in your heart. You can visit there any time to feel the love you deserve. Pain does not exist in the realm of God because it is an illusion, and God is Truth. God is Peace and surely what pain expresses, is conflict. God is Love and He would not have His Son suffer.

In *A Course in Miracles,* Jesus refers to the crucifixion as the last useless sacrifice, meant to be a dramatic lesson about forgiveness. This rang true for me because I know how far reaching sacrifice is. We, and the whole collective mind of humanity, have confused sacrifice, and its incipient pain, with love. We projected onto God that He wanted His Son to sacrifice Himself. How can this be, when sacrifice is a need for pain that is used to compensate for guilt? Sacrifice intends to hide our lack of worth, but only ends up adding to our feelings of valuelessness. It is caught in the vicious circle of superiority-inferiority. Sacrifice is competitive and useless, except to the ego, as anything accomplished by sacrifice could have been accomplished without it. Sacrifice is attack. How could this be God's Will for His Son? If sacrifice does not pass the test of reason, it seems to me that we have projected our belief systems onto God's.

There is at least one tradition that states that, because of His purity, Jesus did not suffer on the cross. Forgiveness equals sinlessness. Sinlessness has no need for pain. As I have studied pain, this made a lot of sense to me.

If we have pain, we are denying God, because we cannot have pain and God at the same time. When it comes to choosing, wouldn't you rather choose God?

Let go of any confusion about God, and your fear. God, who is Love, could only be fearful to your ego. To confuse God with the madness of the world is to think God is mad. The world is our making – the very shadow of our ego.

A Course in Miracles says:

If God is real, there is no pain.

If pain is real, there is no God.

For vengeance is not part of love.

And fear, denying love and using

pain to prove that God is dead, has

shown that death is victor over life.

The body [not the spirit] is the Son of

God, corruptible in death and mortal

as the Father he has slain.

But God is real, and the rest is an illusion of pain. That is why pain can be healed; it is illusion and it does not stand up to truth, order and unity. Attempting to deny God is true madness and it is this madness that leads us to have pain. Our pain is our own hidden desire to crucify another. This is insane. Neither they nor you are guilty, except as you decide. Neither they nor you deserve the savage punishment the mind intends for such crimes. Your belief in your "secret sins," as the Course calls them, is all an illusion and should be treated as such. My experience of close to forty years in the healing profession has proved this to me over and over again.

It is only your mind that condemns you to pain. It is only the illusions you have invested in that could demand such payment. Nothing beyond your thoughts can hurt you or cause you pain. God believes in you enough to know that, sooner or later, you will find your way back to Him, but not through death, which is sleep and keeps you in the same state as when you fell asleep. Finding God comes from awakening. Visit your heart. Find your loving Father. He waits for you. It is not the world that makes you sick or sad. Nothing outside you wounds you, makes you suffer or loses you strength and vitality. Those choices come from the mind, and all else is the agent of the illusions of our mind. Choose with your Loving Father for the truth and for yourself. He Loves You. Let yourself be loved.

Lesson 99 – The Alternative to Pain

Pain is the result of how we see our identity. We view ourselves as a body, and we believe for all the wrong reasons that we deserve punishment. There are no good reasons to punish ourselves unless we wish to reinforce the supposed crime. Guilt is a great reinforcer, as it gives a lot of attention to the mistake, and dark glamour to us. There is an alternative to pain that has to do with our most essential identity and therefore our true one that extends beyond time. This is our identity as a child of God. If we realized our power, we could not think of ourselves as weak and vulnerable. We would have the strength and power of the Universe. We would feel God in our hearts and we would bless the world with that Love. As we broke free of our chains, we would free our brothers and sisters.

If we are God's Child then our last name is God. People who have awakened to higher and higher states of consciousness, experience more and more their oneness with God. But when they reach the highest state of Awakening, there is no more consciousness or dualism, there is only Awareness. At this point in Oneness, enlightened beings speak of themselves as God because all separation has disappeared.

To step out of pain must be God's Will for us, as this is something any loving father would want. And, as any loving father would, He wants us to enjoy our heritage and the legacy that He, as our Father, has provided for us. How much more so does our Father, who waits for us in Oneness, want us to realize our heritage and legacy until we fully realize who we are.

We are the holy child of God Himself, deserving every sweetness and ease. *A Course in Miracles* puts it this way:

"I am the holy Son of God Himself.

I cannot suffer, cannot be in pain;

I cannot suffer loss, nor fail to do

All that salvation asks."

You cannot fail to do what would save you if you were to fully realize these words. If you got the words as truth then everything would change in your world. It would bring a miracle of transformation, not only to your life but to the world itself. Each one who realizes they are the child of God sees the fallacy of death and, from such a high perspective, all of the suffering that proceeds from this belief is also melted away.

You are the holy child of God. All good fortune, all ease and abundance are meant to be yours.

Today, focus on only one thing. You are God's precious child. Let yourself be loved. Let in the grace that would transform your life. You are God's beautiful child and He wishes that you give up being the prodigal child and come home to your feast and your inheritance.

Lesson 100 – Pain is a False Witness

Pain is a false witness to who we think we are, and what we thought we did. We cannot have pain unless we have beliefs about ourselves that have condemned us as wrong, bad, guilty and sinful. Mistakes we made in our lives are dark lessons that can be unlearned. Life is a dream whose only purpose is to learn the lessons that allow us to awaken from the dream. Guilt keeps us locked in the mistake and the pain. What do mistakes count for in a dream? Yet our ego pounces on them as worthy of punishment and continuous torture. This makes the ego strong at heavy cost to ourselves. It reinforces this reality which reflects our ego mind.

In the morning when we awake, we are freed of our dreams. When we awake from the dream of this world, we shall be similarly freed. We shall be in the dream but not of it, in the world but not of it. Our dreams at night express wish fulfillment. Our waking dream, called life, is also an expression of our many conflicting wishes. The guilt that comes from such mistaken and spurious wishes is just a way of cementing over an unlearned lesson with self-attack. If we beat ourselves up for such mistakes in a video game, only the masochistic would play. Life is a full scale video game we play, to learn how to get beyond the video game to Life itself.

The purpose of living this life is to awaken to an ever better way until there is *the Awakening*. We can begin by turning over to God or our Higher Mind every belief we have about ourselves, beliefs in which we think we can suffer and in which we think we deserve suffering. We have condemned ourselves for a crime that is not real, because it is a crime in a dream in which we have come to learn about love. Let us unlearn the mistake we made so that it is replaced with beauty and light. When we correct mistakes in this way we become an agent of innocence and change for those around us.

The perennial philosophies and the old religions of Buddhism and Hinduism see life as a dream. Even the Bible notes that Adam fell into a deep sleep, but nowhere does it say he woke up. To awaken, we must first realize we are asleep and that our experience is a dream experience. Then, in the dream, we must awaken our will, which is our spirit. The dream will continue for us until we awaken and there will be a series of ever greater lessons, meant to be awakenings to joy and a more perfect world as we journey back to the here and now, the nexus of such awakenings. This is why the ego attempts to lose the here and now in pain, which is of the past, and fear which comes of attempting to live in the future.

Since we cannot deal with our own guilt, we project what we thought we did in the dream on others around us and see them as guilty and worthy of punishment. This simply locks us further into the dream. Innocence is a way to awaken and, when we find it inside ourselves, we will find innocence outside ourselves as well, as evidenced by success, abundance, health and love. Otherwise, we toss guilt around like a hot potato, trying to toss it to another before we are burned. And so, we end up keeping it buried within, but attacking another for it.

A *Course in Miracles* speaks of the *secret dream* which is that, in 'the Fall' from Oneness, there was the desire to be separate. Beneath every 'trauma' we had in our lives, there is the secret dream to be separate. Once we discover that we have sold our birthright for an untrue independence, we can begin to reverse this trend as a bad idea whose outcome is pain.

In the dream and in the recesses of the unconscious, we believe that we have attacked that which is unassailable. In our desire to be separate we believe that God has abandoned us and Love is no more. But neither God, nor Love, nor Innocence could abandon us. We could give up our hidden notions of God. We could ask for the truth. We could ask to realize the truth – that it would be impossible for God Who is Love to condemn us. Let us no longer bear false witness against God because nothing can shift Who God is; it can only stop us from receiving His Grace. We have deceived ourselves about ourselves, others and God. We could give up this illusory dream we have made, because what we would wake up to is so much more joy-filled, ordered by truth and touched by beauty.

Summary

Though mystics, quantum physicists or those involved in the transpersonal know the world as a dream, illusion and maya, when anyone suffers, the world seems all too real. Then we need help and when we are ill or in pain anything that seems to help is a godsend. The goal of this book is to be just such a comfort but one that can provide not just a balm but an ongoing sanctuary. While the book is laid out in simple principles; it can be practiced and practiced as we deepen our understanding and develop our thinking into one that promotes healing and is painfree.

When the book is finished, you can pick out a number between 1 and 100 or simply open the book to find your salient lesson for whatever need you find yourself in.

I wish you peace and great good fortune. May you be healthy and happy always and in all ways.

Chuck Spezzano
February 2009
Kahalu'u, Hawai'i